What People Are Saying About
Never Be Sick Again . . .

"Raymond Francis will give you the information you require—and if you combine it with inspiration, self-esteem and self-love, you will accomplish wonders. Take your health into your own hands—choose life and *Never Be Sick Again*!"

—Bernie Siegel, M.D.
author of *Love, Medicine & Miracles*
and *Prescriptions for Living*

"The world is a better place for Raymond Francis and his work. He brings hope and inspiration to those who seek the path out of illness to sustained health and well-being. For the many health mysteries caused by nutritional deficits, overload of toxins and neuro-immuno-hormonal dysfunctions, this book is a necessary and joyful treasure."

—Russ Jaffe, M.D.
fellow, Health Studies Collegium
fellow, National Academy of Clinical Biochemistry

"You must read this inspiring story and learn how one man overcame his own illness to become a fine educator in the science of health maintenance. With our current medical system failing miserably to treat or prevent a wide variety of illnesses, this book is a timely contribution."

—Hyla Cass, M.D.
author of *Natural Highs* and
St. John's Wort: Nature's Blues Buster

Raymond Francis's brush with death as a patient draws the reader to appreciate the lessons he has learned. *Never Be Sick Again* paints a clear picture of the choices that you can make to attain a healthier life. With the skill of a master teacher, he places these choices within reach."

—Richard Kunin, M.D.
president, Society for Orthomolecular Health Medicine
author of *Mega-Nutrition*

"*Never Be Sick Again* presents a revolutionary new understanding of health and disease. Raymond Francis empowers readers and puts them back in charge of their health. This important book offers keen insights into the shifts in thinking about health; it is a prelude to what medicine in the future must become."

—**Al Lemerandé Jr., M.D.**
director of medical programs,
Advanced Physicians Medical Group
author of *Dynamic Health Through Nutrition*

"Reading *Never Be Sick Again* is like learning health in one lesson. This book cuts through the complexity of health and disease with the simple, yet revolutionary, concept of *one disease, two causes and six pathways.* This is future medicine now!"

—**Len Saputo, M.D.**
medical director, Health Medicine Institute

NEVER BE SICK AGAIN

ONE DISEASE • TWO CAUSES • SIX PATHWAYS

HEALTH IS A CHOICE
LEARN HOW TO CHOOSE IT

Raymond Francis, M.Sc.
with Kester Cotton

Foreword by Harvey Diamond
Coauthor of the #1 *NY Times* Bestseller
Fit for Life

Health Communications, Inc.
Deerfield Beach, Florida

www.hci-online.com

Library of Congress Cataloging-in-Publication Data

Francis, Raymond, 1937–
    Never be sick again : Raymond Francis with Kester Cotton ; foreword by Harvey Diamond.
        p. cm.
    ISBN 1-55874-954-3
        1. Health—Miscellanea.   2. Self-care, Health.   3. Healing—Miscellanea.
    4. Health—Philosophy.   5. Mind and body.   I. Cotton, Kester.   II. Title.

RA776.5 .F736 2002
613—dc21

                                                                    2002033399

Publisher: Health Communications, Inc.
                3201 S.W. 15th Street
                Deerfield Beach, FL 33442-8190

R-08-03

Cover design by Larissa Hise Henoch
Inside design by Lisa Camp and Dawn Von Strolley Grove

CONTENTS

FOREWORD

N ever Be Sick Again takes the mystery out of disease. This groundbreaking book presents a revolutionary theory of health and disease: There are not thousands of different diseases, but only one disease: malfunctioning cells. Put simply, if the cells that make up your body are healthy, then you are healthy. Take care of your cells by providing them with all the nutrients they need, keep them free of injurious toxins, and disease will not happen. That concept is what this book is all about.

Never Be Sick Again is health made simple, written by someone who figured it out the hard way. In 1985, author Raymond Francis (a chemist and a graduate of MIT) suffered a near-fatal health condition. He used his knowledge of biochemistry to save his own life, and during his recovery, Francis asked himself fundamental questions like, "Why do people get sick?" and, "How can disease be prevented or reversed?" The answers to these questions are the essence of Francis's new theory: *One disease, two causes* of disease and *six pathways* between health and disease. Explained in easy-to-understand language, this concept of health and disease is scientifically grounded in cutting-edge cellular biochemistry and molecular biology. *Never Be Sick Again* is the distilled wisdom of hundreds of books, thousands of scientific journals and over sixteen years of experience and observation. Francis's book provides a simple and holistic approach that can help to prevent and/or reverse almost any disease—the ultimate triumph over disease.

A book like this is needed now more than ever. Health-care costs continue to rise while the health of the American people continues to decline. The average person is lost in a glut of complex and confusing health information. When we do get sick, though, not understanding why we are sick or how to become well, we feel like powerless victims, subject to seemingly random infections and genetic predispositions. We feel helpless because our understanding of disease remains stuck in the archaic germ theory. We worry too much about our bodies being invaded by microorganisms and not enough about building and maintaining the overall health and function of our cells. Disease is not a random event. We can choose to prevent it, provided that we know how. Health is determined by what we, as individuals, are willing to do for ourselves; it is our responsibility.

Rather than being a game of chance, health is a choice. Whether we realize it or not, the daily choices we make have a direct impact on the health of our cells. When we make the wrong choices, and our health takes a turn for the worse, we blame genes or germs or the aging process rather than the way we live our lives. In truth, the only way to heal any disease is to normalize cellular function by correcting cellular malfunction, the common denominator of all disease.

Modern medicine has a poor understanding of disease and relies on suppressing the symptoms of disease rather than addressing its true causes. Little wonder most of us die from chronic and degenerative diseases—such as cancer and heart disease—that are "treated" but seldom healed. As a society, our applying the principles of the six pathways outlined in this book is crucial. Doing so will improve the health of our population to where most of existing medical practice can become irrelevant. Even now when we recognize the existence of only one disease, breaking medicine up into medical specialties becomes obsolete and counterproductive.

Raymond Francis provides real answers for real life, regardless of who you are or your state of health. By providing a powerful framework for maintaining optimal health, this book ties all the basics together in a way that anyone can put to immediate and practical use. Francis simplifies the health equation to the lowest common denominator—each individual cell. If you take care of each cell in your body, disease cannot happen.

An island of clarity in a sea of confusion, *Never Be Sick Again* is a one-stop solution for health professionals and laymen alike. Think of this book as health in one lesson. Everyone, especially our children, should learn about this cutting-edge approach to health and disease. In the past, health and disease have seemed like mysteries over which we have little control, but no longer. Now, we do have control. Knowing of just one disease and only two causes of disease gives us the power to get well and stay well. Francis's title says it all: *Never Be Sick Again*.

Harvey Diamond
coauthor of the #1 *New York Times* bestseller, *Fit for Life*

ACKNOWLEDGMENTS

N o one works in isolation; the seventeen-year journey that led up to this book attests to that. I have many individuals to thank, in addition to my wonderful publisher Health Communications, Inc., for making *Never Be Sick Again* a reality. I want to express my gratitude to the great thinkers who came before me and upon whose work I have built, pioneers such as Hippocrates, Claude Bernard, Antoine Bechamp, René Dubos, Alexis Carrel, Hans Selye, Walter Cannon, Linus Pauling, Roger Williams, Emanuel Cheraskin and many others. I want to thank my professors and colleagues at M.I.T., who helped to sharpen my critical thinking skills. I want to thank Dr. Russell Jaffe, who pointed me in the right direction as I was searching for answers to my questions about health and disease.

Many thanks to my mother and father for their love and for helping me to become who I am. Many thanks to my family and friends for their encouragement and for the many hours they spent reading and commenting on various drafts of chapters. In particular, I would like to gratefully acknowledge

Mark Baird, David Buttaro, Joan Carole, Br. Camillus Chavez, Mark Choquet, Kathleen Cotton, Peter DeTomi, Bernard Friesecke, Pascal Girard, Dr. Peter Litchfield, Kathleen Martuza, Robert Menkemeller, Mollie Meyers, Dr. David Rovno, Brandon Soule, Pamela Strong, Nancy Talbot, and Alec Wilson, who helped to make this book more understandable and useful to the reader. Thanks also to my two wonderful editors, Linda Hall and Beatrice Trum Hunter, who contributed so much to making this a better book.

I am also grateful for the hundreds of people I have worked with as a health advisor. Each and every one of them taught me something important about health and helped to cement my understanding of the importance of diet and lifestyle in preventing and reversing disease.

Last, but far from least, I would like to thank my cowriter Kester Cotton. Without your support, there would be no book to read. Thank you for your friendship, encouragement, patience, forbearance and years of hard work. The days we have spent creating *Never Be Sick Again* will always be cherished memories.

INTRODUCTION

I was too sick to leave my bed. In fact, I was too weak even to lift my head from the pillow. At age forty-eight, at the peak of an international business career, I found myself on the brink of death. I had lost forty pounds from an already thin frame; I looked skeletal. My vital signs were failing. My doctors expected me to die.

I chose to live. I say "chose" because on my own, relying on my knowledge of biochemistry and my determination not to die, I saved my own life. I took some fairly simple steps, but I also took one profound leap. I made a powerful discovery: *Almost all disease can be prevented or reversed. As a result, health is a choice and no one has to be sick.*

This book presents an entirely new theory of health and disease that will ultimately change the way medicine is practiced. This book offers a revolutionary way to perceive health, a guidebook for living based on cutting-edge science that is simple to understand. This guide gives you the power to control your own health in a way that you perhaps never imagined possible.

In reality, humans experience only one disease. *All disease is the result of malfunctioning cells,* no matter if the disease is a "common" cold, a mental illness such as depression or a life-threatening cancer. This theory of malfunctioning cells cuts through the confusion of health and disease and provides a unifying understanding of what keeps people well or makes them sick.

The two causes of disease, the two reasons that cells malfunction, are *deficiency* (insufficient nutrients) and *toxicity* (excessive toxins). These two causes work through six areas of daily life: the six pathways each person travels toward health or disease. If you take care of your body's needs along these six pathways, you give your cells what they need and you avoid what is toxic. You will not become sick.

The theory presented in this book—a unifying theory of disease—is the most important health discovery to emerge in the last few hundred years. No such theory existed during the evolution of what we now call "modern medicine," which explains why the medical establishment cannot cure nor prevent disease as effectively as it might. My theory of health offers power, simplicity and clarity in place of powerlessness, which is what most people now feel. Most people are overwhelmed and confused by the constant flood of conflicting health information, the thousands of different diseases that physicians "treat" with drugs and surgery. This swirl of specialists, symptoms and side effects leaves people without cures for their disease and, too often, either growing sicker or facing death. We end up powerless because we have no idea why we are sick or how to make ourselves well again.

My new approach asks you to make profound shifts in what has been conventional thinking about illness and health care. By preventing and reversing disease through the six pathways, you put the power to get better and stay well into *your* hands. If you are so sick that you have given up hope, this approach is the light of choice. Had I this level of understanding years ago, I would never have become sick in the first place.

I have shared my ideas with thousands of people around the world, including hundreds of medical doctors. I have seen people who have been sick for a decade or more apply this information and quickly become well again. I have seen people who have fruitlessly tried endless doctors, hospitals, clinics, medications and even gimmicks. They become well again by applying logical, sound, scientific approaches to enhancing health at the cellular level.

This book asks you to think outside the box of traditional medicine—a box that may have you stifled by misinformation and cut off from the kind of understanding that will truly make you well. Consider how conventional thinking can trap us: Why do we easily accept that stress can make us sick, but we have difficulty embracing the idea that love, laughter and a balanced life can make us well? Why are we willing to ingest chemicals in the form of prescription drugs that are alien to our body, but we are skeptical that natural substances—primarily the right foods—can heal? Why are we willing to recognize the damage of an obvious poisoning—a major chemical spill, for instance—but we ignore the devastating effects of small amounts of toxic substances, which accumulate in our bodies and make us a little bit sicker every day?

Our bodies have an amazing capacity to heal, but they are more vulnerable than you may realize. This book teaches you how to tap that capacity for healing and how to avoid the toxins and the stresses—in the environment and inside your own body—that make you sick. Many dangers around us go unrecognized, but they take a toll every day.

My theory of wellness takes you to the front lines of the battle between health and disease: the cell. Your body is made up of trillions of cells. Cells have needs, which I identify, that must be met if they are to function well. If your cells are healthy, your body will not become sick. If your cells do not receive what they need or if they are damaged or poisoned, they will stop working right and you will become sick. (You may be surprised to discover what is toxic to your cells.) Cells that receive what they need and avoid harm can function well and provide for healthy life, regardless of your age, the genes you have inherited or the "germs" to which you have been exposed. Healthy cells refuse disease; no one with healthy cells has any reason to become sick, not even to contract a cold. People alive today are far sicker than most of us recognize, and they die decades sooner than their genetic potential. Healthy life, well past one hundred years old, should be our birthright.

We do not usually think about health in this way. We don't knowingly choose disease, but we do choose diets and lifestyles that lead to disease. Unable to predict, prevent or conquer disease, most people and most physicians pursue treatment—such as prescription or over-the-counter drugs—once obvious symptoms have presented, after massive cellular malfunction has already occurred. Patients and their physicians treat body parts or body systems as unrelated. The mainstream medical community has no unifying theory of disease, no unifying treatment and no plan for prevention, and therefore true and lasting health is an illusion.

This book describes how to keep your body—all your cells—truly healthy. Understanding the six pathways toward health and following them in the right direction will change your life. You will learn things about nutrition that you have probably never heard before, including how the way you shop, the way you cook or the foods that you combine at a meal spell the difference between health and disease. You will learn to recognize hazards in your home and how to stop toxins from being *created* within your own body.

You'll learn specifics, down to the kind of vitamin supplements you should take, the toothpaste you should use and the olive oil you should buy. I name names and identify brands based on how the products affect cells, because buying the wrong products does nothing to keep you healthy. Certain products, in fact, make you unhealthy.

Consider your own life: Do you suffer from a health condition that you have given up trying to cure and now accept as fate? Do you bounce from one medical specialist to another, dizzy with conflicting diagnoses and different ideas about which treatments are best? Is your cabinet full of medications that you take regularly without any sense that you are healing? Are you tired most of the time? Do you expect to live past your eighties?

This book guides you out of the maze of medical specialists and on a path toward wellness. This book teaches you how to question your doctors' advice and how to evaluate, on your own, the medicines you should take, if any. You can regain the kind of energy for living that you may have thought was lost forever. With this book you can learn how to live beyond one hundred years of age.

By looking at health and disease in entirely new ways, and understanding how to choose health, you can reevaluate illnesses that you may have come to accept as unavoidable. You may be shocked to discover how often you choose not to be healthy. My code for living shows you, in big ways and in small ways, how to stop making yourself sick. I describe a potential for human health—and long life—that you never thought possible. Horizons will open up as you consider the possibility that you can live, fully and vigorously, decades beyond what you now consider old age.

Many people know more about how their automobiles work than about what their bodies need in order to function, and people often pay more attention to maintaining their cars than themselves. People feel they just don't have the knowledge or medical training to figure out what is wrong with their own bodies or how to heal. The truth is that knowledge and power are within one's reach. No theory about health is so simple yet so powerful. This approach clears up the confusion surrounding thousands of so-called "diseases," and eliminates most modern medical treatments—drugs and surgery—as toxic, invasive and rarely necessary. The focus, instead, is on the common problems of disease and how to solve them. This book bypasses the complex and confusing world of illness and remedies and simplifies our understanding of health and disease, enabling people to prevent and reverse disease by addressing its causes. From the tangle of all the complexity emerges a straightforward approach to becoming well and staying well—an island of clarity in a sea of confusion.

In its simplest terms, how health is determined can be expressed as an equation:

Health = positive things minus negative things

The quality of your health is determined by the positive things you do *for* your body minus the negative things you do *to* your body. This concept is not complicated, sexy or original; it is simply the truth. The problem is that accurate information about the factors that affect this equation is hard to obtain. Accurate information about what is positive and good for you and what is not does not come easily. Contradictory information and myths circulate, and people disseminate opinions as if they were facts. Many health writers, untrained in science, misinterpret scientific information or parrot each other. The blind are often leading the blind. To choose health, you must know how to distinguish between good choices and bad choices regarding diet, toxic exposure, exercise, prescription and recreational drug use, stress and other factors. This book shows you how to make these distinctions.

You may already read the labels on the foods you buy, the warnings on the prescriptions you take and the coverage limits of your health plan, but if you are to achieve health and stay healthy, you must first understand what your body needs. Many health books provide recipes, diet lists, exercise regimens and the like—routines to be blindly followed with no real understanding of the rationale behind them. This book is different. This book provides a powerful and logical conception of health, a framework that assists you in coming to your own conclusions and making your own choices. With this framework, you will have a basis for understanding which choices need to be made, when you should make them and why.

Your body is made of cells. When a large number of your cells malfunction, body systems become disrupted, leading to *cellular malfunction*. Cellular malfunction has only *two causes*: *deficiency*, cells not getting what they need, and *toxicity*, cells poisoned by something they do not need. Finally, *six pathways* exist between health and disease through which the health of our cells can change for better or worse. We can become healthy or sick (i.e., deficient and/or toxic) through the following pathways:

- Pathway 1—Nutrition

  You are what you eat. Learn how to select and prepare the types of foods that will enable your cells to function at their best.

- Pathway 2—Toxin

  A toxin is a substance that interferes with normal cellular function, thereby causing malfunction, which is disease. Learn where toxins are found and how you can avoid them.

- Pathway 3—Psychological

  The body and mind are inseparably connected; they are one and the same thing. The way we react to life events and respond to our thoughts and emotions directly affect our cells.

- Pathway 4—Physical

  Our cells and bodies need physical maintenance, like an automobile. Do you have enough exercise, rest, sunlight and fresh air?

- Pathway 5—Genetic

  Genes affect our cells, but not nearly as much as modern medicine would have us believe. Learn how to optimize your genetic potential and avoid genetic damage.

- Pathway 6—Medical

  Modern medicine kills and injures millions of people every year. Learn how medicine affects your cells, and make educated decisions about which treatments you need and which you do not.

All you need to know at any point in time is in which direction you are going along each of the pathways—toward health or disease—and to make corrections. You cannot make good choices along only one or two of the pathways and expect to achieve optimal health; this approach limits many health plans and books, useful though they may be. Many approaches are on the right track, but they do not look at the whole picture. Making healthy choices with respect to all six pathways is what empowers the body to regulate and repair itself.

That said, each choice you make in a positive direction, toward health, on any pathway at any time will improve your life. Each step toward health puts you closer to your true potential and further away from the risk of disease or illness. Each contribution, no matter how small, is still significant.

1

I ALMOST DIED

One Disease

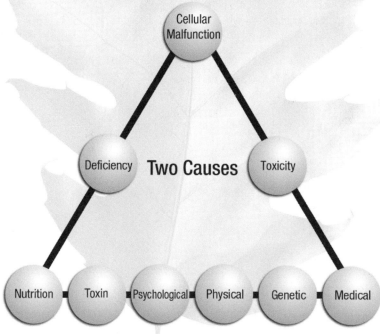

Cellular Malfunction

Deficiency **Two Causes** Toxicity

Nutrition | Toxin | Psychological | Physical | Genetic | Medical

Six Pathways

"The next major advance in the health of the American people will be determined by what the individual is willing to do for himself."

John Knowles
former president, The Rockefeller Foundation

Not too many years ago, no one would have been able to convince me that I would be writing a definitive book about human health and performance. I was no health expert; in fact, I gave little thought to the subject. I assumed I was healthy and that I could do little to improve upon it. Yet, here I am today, devoting my life to researching and improving health.

Concern for our health is something we all have in common. We all would like to live a high-quality, disease-free life, no matter how long that life may be. But most of us have no idea that a disease-free life is possible, so our priorities become out of whack, and we form habits that jeopardize our health. Then we ignore the early signs of ill health and, without knowing it, we lay the groundwork for disaster. That is exactly what I did.

At the height of my former career, I was president of an

international management consulting firm specializing in international competitiveness, industrial quality and productivity. I was a consultant to Fortune 500 companies, the State Department, the United Nations and to the prime ministers of several foreign governments. Life had been good to me.

Then the early warning signs that things were changing came in 1983. I began to slow down, requiring more sleep and tiring more easily. I began to experience frequent allergic reactions, including runny nose, itchy eyes, sneezing, heart palpitations and skin rashes. I suffered muscle aches and joint pain. I felt as though I was losing my edge, losing some of the mental and physical capacity that had allowed me to operate at the highest levels of international business and government. Life was becoming less fun and more like a chore.

I brought these complaints to the attention of my physician, a man who the medical community rated as "one of the best." He examined me, did many tests and pronounced me in "excellent health." When I protested, saying I did not feel like I was in excellent health, he replied, "You are just getting older." I protested again, saying that in my whole life I had never felt this way before. He continued, "Well, you have never been this old before." I was forty-six years old.

I would later discover that physicians have no protocols or established procedures for measuring early decline in health. Instead they blame "getting older" for so many feelings of ill health, even at ages when human beings have the potential to be in their prime (remember, I was only forty-six when I began suffering from problems attributed to my age). Physicians consistently assume that the patient is "well" until his or her condition deteriorates into symptoms that the doctor recognizes as a diagnosable disease.

Over the next year and a half, my symptoms worsened. My fatigue became more pronounced; I required ever-increasing amounts of sleep, and even then I felt tired. The fatigue made it increasingly difficult to travel, as my job required. My allergic reactions were becoming more severe. I would experience sneezing fits so dramatic that I would have to rest after them. My heart palpitations were more frequent and pronounced. I would see colored rings around lights and my vision would blur.

I finally decided to seek the assistance of an allergy specialist. Little did I realize, as I entered the doctor's office that fateful morning, that it would be the last day of life as I had known it. The allergist administered a diagnostic test called an intradermal test, whereby an allergen is injected into the skin with a hypodermic needle. The procedure is much more provocative and sensitive than the typical scratch tests familiar to most people. Intradermal tests may identify allergies that might otherwise be missed. However, if someone is especially sensitive to an allergen, this type of test can provoke a serious reaction. My doctor neglected to tell me that the FDA regularly receives reports of injuries and deaths from these tests. My condition and the fact that I was experiencing significant allergic reactions at the time should have prompted this physician to be more cautious and anticipate that an intradermal test might provoke a serious reaction.

It did.

The reaction was catastrophic, causing my immune system to spin out of control. During the next week I slept almost constantly and appeared to have aged about ten years. I suffered fatigue and disability unlike anything I had ever experienced. Prior to the test, although I had some serious allergy problems, I was still able to function relatively normally; afterward, I was seriously ill and almost completely dysfunctional.

Years later, another physician—one considerably better informed—gave me a meaningful description of what had happened to me. He described my state of compromised health as rather like standing on the edge of a precipice. My allergist did not recognize my vulnerability and the need to work initially with nutritional support and conservative treatments to back me away from that edge. The allergist's decision to administer a provocative test pushed me off the precipice and into an abyss of catastrophic health decline.

Ten months later, I was still in that abyss of illness and anxiety, with my health in a downward spiral. In the past, whenever I had been sick, I had always recovered in a matter of days or weeks. This time was different indeed. I experienced chronic fatigue, multiple chemical sensitivities and allergic reactions to almost everything. I also developed several autoimmune syndromes, including Sjogren's syndrome, Hashimoto's thyroiditis and lupus. In these syndromes, the immune system attacks the body's own tissues, causing a cascade of serious problems. In my case, my immune system was attacking my salivary glands, lachrymal glands, thyroid gland, kidneys and connective tissue. I had an extensive list of debilitating symptoms including dizziness, impaired memory, depression, heart palpitations, blurred vision, muscle and joint pain, diarrhea, bloating, nausea, numbness and even seizures. I was unable to perform any meaningful activity. My health was gone, and life, as I had known it, was over.

During those ten nightmarish months, I visited thirty-six medical doctors. I had so many different symptoms that I was referred to specialists for each one, including ophthalmologists, gastroenterologists, neurologists, endocrinologists, cardiologists, allergists, rheumatologists, psychiatrists, internists and immunologists. Being bounced from one specialist to another, sometimes seeing two or even three in a day, was very frustrating. I certainly heard plenty of second, third and fourth opinions, often conflicting, but none particularly helpful. My multitude of symptoms totally baffled those learned specialists. (How much easier it would have been had they known what I know now: that there is only one disease and that symptoms are not important.) They performed many expensive diagnostic tests, which served little purpose other than to give fancy names to my symptoms, such as neuropathy, colitis, arrhythmia, arthralgia, keratitis sicca, thyroiditis and others.

They were merely describing my symptoms with a technical name, the usual diagnosing, and then sending a bill. A few suggested that I was a hypochondriac, imagining ill health. Many physicians assume that if they do not understand what is wrong, the patient must be imagining his illness. At the time, I thought all of my doctors were baffled because my case was so complex. In the end, however, the answers proved to be simple. The answers had been there all along. One just needed to know where to look.

From Bad to Worse

As sick as I was after ten months of illness, things were about to become much worse. One of the last physicians I went to see made a decision that nearly killed me. He prescribed an antiparasitic drug, metronidazole, which turned out to be heptatoxic (poisonous to the liver). I suffered a severe reaction to the drug. In my weakened and chemically sensitive condition I should never have been given this drug, as I would later learn from the medical literature. Perhaps I should have known better, given my prior experiences with medical doctors, but trusting the doctor and knowing of no other options, I took the drug. Metronidazole is known to be stressful to the liver, and my liver was already under a lot of stress. I could not handle the additional toxic load. My liver failed, and I was at death's door.

As I lay in bed, deathly ill with chemical hepatitis, my weight dropped from an already trim 160 pounds (at 6-foot-2) to a positively skeletal 120. I was too weak even to lift my head. My vital signs were failing, and my physicians doubted that I would survive. Death appeared certain.

Had I continued to rely on conventional medicine, I would not be here today, and you would not be reading my story. As weak as I was, something inside of me was not ready to let go—not without a fight. But I did not know where to turn for help. As I look back, I am amazed at the chain of events that saved my life and allowed me to regain control of my health.

My brother, bless his heart, started the process. During my illness, he had flown across the country to be with me. He gave me a book that proved instrumental in saving my life: Norman Cousins's bestseller, *Anatomy of an Illness*. In 1964, Norman Cousins, a layman with no medical or scientific training, was diagnosed with ankylosing spondylitis, a connective tissue disease that deteriorates collagen (the "glue" that holds our cells together). Cousins's disease was literally causing his body to fall apart. His illness, like mine, was deemed by his physicians to be incurable and fatal. Unwilling to accept such a prognosis, Cousins sought whatever knowledge he could to help himself. He succeeded. Not only did he find ways to save his own life; he later became a professor of medicine at UCLA.

Cousins took action in four areas. First, like myself, Cousins recognized that he was being harmed by his medical treatment. He concluded that the drugs his physicians were prescribing were so toxic that they were accelerating his decline. He stopped taking the drugs. Second, he discovered the enormous power of the mind over the body. The excruciating pain he was experiencing was affected by his attitude toward the pain. By learning to change his attitude, he could reduce his pain. Third, he found laughter to be helpful; ten minutes of genuine, hearty laughter would cause his pain to go away for hours. He started watching funny movies, and when the effect would wear off, he would switch on the projector and laugh some more. The laughter had profound and beneficial effects on his body chemistry and contributed to his recovery. Fourth, he discovered the powerful anti-inflammatory properties of vitamin C. He decided to take twenty-five grams a day administered by intravenous drip. This action had a profoundly beneficial effect on his highly inflammatory condition. By avoiding toxic prescription drugs, changing his attitude, laughing and administering plenty of vitamin C, Cousins made a miraculous recovery.

Lying on what had been pronounced my deathbed, I thought about Cousins's book in relation to my graduate school days doing scientific research at MIT. I wondered how Cousins managed to find the pertinent information he needed to save himself. If Cousins, a dying man with no scientific training, could obtain such critical, life-saving knowledge, why couldn't his physicians? After all, these professionals had devoted their entire careers to medicine. Knowing that Cousins had found a way to save his own life encouraged me; I hoped that my scientific training as a chemist might enable me to do the same.

As I lay there with a poisoned liver, dying from chemical hepatitis, I realized that if I wanted to live I must act quickly. Not much time was left. Thinking about how instrumental vitamin C was in Cousins's recovery, I remembered from my study of biochemistry that vitamin C plays an essential role in liver detoxification. Because my liver had been poisoned by a toxic drug, perhaps some vitamin C would help it detoxify. It seemed like an experiment worth doing, and besides, I knew of no other options.

It worked.

Twenty-four hours after starting oral doses of vitamin C (about four grams a day), my vital signs began to stabilize. In forty-eight hours I was able to sit up in bed. A few days before, death had been a certainty. Now, I could sit up, which was the first time I had experienced a measurable improvement in all those months. Progress, even in the form of something as simple as sitting up in bed, can be incredibly inspiring. At that point, I knew I could take action that would make a difference. Meanwhile, my physicians could not understand why I not only survived but actually improved.

I was still far from well, though. I was a frail skeleton. I had difficulty performing the simplest tasks, such as dressing, or tying my shoelaces. I had no energy and became fatigued from the slightest exertion. My hands and feet were numb; I had difficulty walking and moved slowly. I was lightheaded and tended to fall over easily. Worse, my brain had trouble functioning; I felt like I was in a mental fog. I had difficulty with short-term memory and simple calculations. Even as I improved enough to venture out again, I could not make correct change at the grocery store and easily forgot what I intended to do.

Perhaps worst of all was the horrific chemical sensitivity that I continued to suffer, causing me to become weak, disoriented and debilitated. The toxic assault on my body by the metronidazole had left me with acute chemical sensitivities. For instance, when I turned on a water faucet the subtle chlorine fumes coming out with the water were enough to cause me to become weak, lightheaded and disoriented. I could not read or be near printed materials because of the chemical fumes coming from the ink and paper. I used only a speakerphone because I would react to the fumes off-gassing from the plastic telephone receiver. My gas water heater had to be replaced with an electric unit because I reacted to the combustion fumes diffusing into the surrounding living space. I had to wear clothes made only from natural fibers, to avoid the toxic fumes from synthetics. I had to purchase special water and air filters. But even with these many precautions, I was debilitated by my relentless reactions to a myriad of environmental chemicals.

Someone who has not personally experienced chemical sensitivity has a hard time understanding how just a whiff of certain chemicals can create total havoc in a matter of seconds. I remember once taking a piece of Scotch tape off a roll and being devastated for the rest of the day by the seemingly inconsequential chemical odor from the tape! With chemical sensitivity, the nervous system develops a "memory" of past reactions. This effect is called *classical conditioning* (i.e., biological learning) and upon detecting these reactive agents again, even in infinitesimal quantities, a full-scale response is produced. Our modern world is permeated with chemicals that can produce such reactions in susceptible people.

In this hideous state of health, I fell into a deep depression. I thought about taking my life. Although I had made some progress, I was allergic to almost everything, and I was in a constant state of debilitating reactions. My life was ruined. No doctor could help me. I was unable to do any meaningful activity and had nothing to look forward to. I could not even watch television because of the chemical fumes off-gassing from the TV set as it heated up.

Choosing to Live

One beautiful afternoon, I was sitting out in the sun and contemplating the meaning of life. Illness has a powerful way of providing perspective and time to think about the really important things. I asked myself whether or not I wanted to continue living. I decided that I did not want to die—I wanted to live. However, life was not worth living in such a debilitated state. My only option was to find a way to become healthy again.

How could I do this? The doctors could not help. In large measure, doctors had brought me to my failing condition. I recall thinking about the explosion of knowledge in the world—about all the new scientific data being published every day. Surely somewhere, some key bit of information would help me. I became determined to find out whatever I could, but it was not easy. My vision was blurred and my eyes hurt. Given that I was unable to be near printed materials because of the ink fumes, how could I study? My mind didn't work right, either: Contemporary literature about chemically sensitive people describes this debilitating type of "brain fog." In my early quests to research my health condition, I would find myself lost in a mental fog, spending hours reading the same material repeatedly without realizing it. Ironically, I was reacting to the very materials I was using to learn how to restore my health.

Still, I remained determined. I purchased a respirator mask to protect me from the chemicals coming from the ink in my study materials. Unfortunately, the rubber part of the mask gave off toxic fumes. I took the mask apart, boiled the rubber pieces in water for two days and then reassembled it, which made the mask tolerable so I could wear it while I did the necessary work.

Next, I purchased a portable electric oven and one hundred feet of outdoor extension cord. I placed the oven downwind from my house and baked all of my reading materials in order to drive off the ink chemicals. Bizarre, but it worked. Now at least I could handle and read my rapidly accumulating piles of medical and scientific literature. I began to educate myself, looking for clues that might help to restore and improve my health.

Thus began a new phase of my life, which continues to this day.

I came across fascinating information as I searched for the answers to my questions. I read technical papers written by a biochemist who, like myself, had become chemically hypersensitive. No physician had been able to help him either, and his sensitivity was so great that he was forced to move to a distant location that harbored no man-made chemicals. He moved into a small wooden shack on a remote beach. Eventually, through his understanding of biochemistry, he was able to take steps to restore his health.

Knowing that someone else had been able to heal himself of this horrendous condition gave me the hope I needed so much. His example convinced me that I, too, would be able to help myself to understand the biochemistry of my illness and apply sound scientific principles to solve my problems. It took me two years of learning and experimenting to raise myself from the depths of liver failure, chronic fatigue, autoimmune diseases and chemical hypersensitivity. Recovery took a great deal of persistence, willingness to try new things and acceptance of many setbacks.

In particular at the height of my chemical sensitivities, I had to be extremely careful about the products I selected. Even minute amounts of toxins were enough to make me ill. I ended up with a kitchen full of vitamin supplements that I could not take because of toxic impurities and my level of susceptibility. Even healthy people are harmed by these impurities, though it may not be as evident to them.

I learned the hard way how suffering can come when health is failing, and when you try remedies that do more harm than good. Even with my scientific training, finding the answers was difficult. Particularly with vitamin supplements and personal care products, a great deal of conflicting information abounds, and consumers remain confused about how to make the best choices. Accurate health information is in great demand, and that is precisely what this book provides. I want to share what I have learned about getting well and staying well.

In 1991, I resigned from all my business and community activities and devoted myself to teaching others how to be healthy. I started by speaking to groups—at first, the same support groups to which I had belonged during the depths of my illness. Then I branched out with a wider audience, which evolved into a regular evening workshop series that continued for years. Later, a publisher became aware of my work and invited me to write a column for his newspaper. After that, I started a radio show called *An Ounce of Prevention* and began publishing my own newsletter, *Beyond Health News*. This book is the next step.

Reaching Our Potential

One of the most profound conclusions I have reached is that *health is a choice;* virtually no one ever has to be sick. The potential for human health and longevity is far greater than we are now achieving. Scientific studies describe populations who lived longer and healthier lives than we do, simply because their societies made dietary and lifestyle choices that supported human health. With just a little knowledge and effort, we can do the same. We can choose health, but first we must educate ourselves.

My own quest for an understanding of how the body maintains and heals itself continues to this day. Throughout my research, I continue to ask myself basic questions, such as:

- What is health?
- What is disease?
- Why do people get sick?
- How can disease be prevented or reversed?
- How long can people live in good health, and what does it take to achieve this?
- What is the potential for human health and longevity?

Please allow me to pass on to you a truly revolutionary theory of health and disease, one that is so simple and powerful that it gives you the choice to never be sick again.

2

YOUR POTENTIAL FOR HEALTH

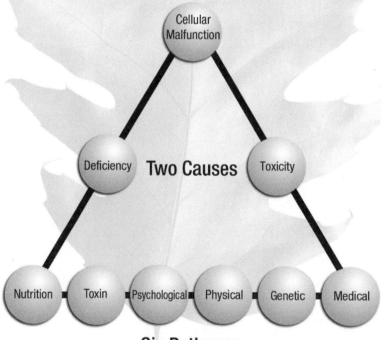

One Disease

Cellular Malfunction

Deficiency   Two Causes   Toxicity

Nutrition   Toxin   Psychological   Physical   Genetic   Medical

Six Pathways

"There is no reason in the world why over 75 percent of the American people should be suffering from degenerative and deficiency diseases. Disease never comes without a cause. If a person is sick and ailing it is because he has been doing something wrong. He needs an education in how to live a healthy life."

Jay M. Hoffman, Ph.D.

Hunza

Most people expect to be sick at least one or more times each year, to cope with at least one serious illness by midlife, and in all likelihood, to die of one or several diseases by their eighties, if not sooner. Most people also think poor health is mainly the result of bad luck and that their longevity is a matter of good fortune.

Nothing could be further from the truth. Poor health is not a matter of luck; poor health is a matter of choice. We do not "get" sick. We make ourselves sick by making bad choices and, conversely, we get healthy and stay healthy by making good ones. Most people feel that they are "healthy" as long as they have no symptoms of disease. Few people realize what optimal health really feels like—and even fewer accept the notion that a vigorous and healthy life beyond 100 years old is within reach. In reality, that kind of long life is what we should all routinely expect.

Meet the face of optimal health. His name is Jose Maria Roa, and he is 131 years old. Jose lives with his family in a small village, high in the Andes Mountains of Ecuador. While his face is weatherworn, his mind is keen, his heart is healthy, his teeth are strong and the lines around his face are born of smiles and the joy of a loving wife and family. Still working on his small farm every day and enjoying an active sex life, Jose fathered his last child at the age of 107. When asked if he'd ever been sick, he replied, "Yes, I have been." Jose had a few colds—that's it—in 131 years! Until his death at 137, Jose remained in perfect health.

Surely this is not normal. Isn't Jose a medical miracle, an aberration of nature? Not so. In his remote village, Jose's health and longevity are far from unusual explains Morton Walker, D.P.M., whose 1985 book *Secrets of Long Life* is based on his study of these hardy people native to the Vilcabamba Valley. For instance, in his queries to the Vilcabambans about the mental health of their society, Walker asked if the older people suffered memory loss due to dementia. These long-lived people had never experienced anything like dementia. They didn't understand the question and, in fact, did not even have words in their language to describe such a condition. Meanwhile, we are told that dementia is a disease of aging and the price we must pay for our so-called "longevity." As I studied Jose—and people like him—I began to understand the potential that all humans have to be healthy.

In America today, we are usually told—and believe—that illnesses like cancer, arthritis, dementia, osteoporosis, diabetes and heart disease are "diseases of aging," but these chronic conditions are not the inevitable result of growing older. Rather, they are the inevitable result of living lifestyles that cannot support human health. In America today, these conditions are epidemic. Having achieved enormous advances in science and medicine, why are we experiencing the largest epidemic of chronic disease in human history?

As I studied patterns of health and disease, I made a profound discovery. I learned that disease does not just randomly happen; it occurs for specific reasons. We are not typically perfectly healthy until we "get" sick, nor does perfect health return once disease has run its course. Although we tend to perceive life this way, the distinctions between health and disease are far less black and white. Remember your cells. Only after massive numbers of cells malfunction or die do you begin to notice symptoms of disease. In other words, you are already sick before you "get sick." People who are truly healthy do not "get sick."

If you stop to consider what it might be like to live in good health to a ripe old age, everything begins to seem different. This potential for health can be described as *optimal* health, where your cells are functioning as well as they possibly can. This level of health is almost guaranteed to keep disease at bay.

A Poor Record

Very few Americans grow old in good health and die naturally from the aging process. Instead, we get sick and die from entirely preventable diseases such as cancer, heart disease, stroke and diabetes. Preventing these health problems is simple, and I will teach you how to do it, but first realize how dire our health problems really are.

The United States spends far more on health, in total and per capita, than any other nation in the world, but our overall health still ranks quite poorly. According to the World Health Organization (WHO), the United States ranks thirty-seventh in overall health quality. It should serve as a wake-up call for all Americans when a third-world country like Oman spends only $334 per person per year on health and ranks eighth in the world, while the United States spends more than ten times that much and we are thirty-seventh. Considering what we spend on health care, shouldn't we be the healthiest nation on Earth? We are not.

People in their teens or early twenties should be at peak levels of health, right? Not in our society. Autopsies performed on accident victims of this age group in Los Angeles revealed that nearly 80 percent had early stages of heart disease; 15 percent had arteries that were more than half blocked. Had these young people survived, they would likely have been victims of a stroke or heart attack. They may have appeared healthy and lived normal lives, but they were definitely not healthy.

It's a matter of perspective. *Our own ill health does not stand out when compared to our unhealthy friends and neighbors.* The allergies, the colds, the flu, the arthritis, the premature aging—all of these seem perfectly normal. Because it is so common in our society, we have come to believe that disease is an inevitable, natural, "normal" part of the aging process.

We mistake being able to function for being healthy. We perceive "sick" as being bedridden or housebound, and "healthy" as being able to go about our normal activities. Healthy does not merely mean being ambulatory and free of obvious disease symptoms. *Healthy means functioning at the highest level that genetic capacity allows.* As in other areas of life, recognizing and admitting the problem is half the battle. Unfortunately, we are a sick population, growing sicker by the day and, worse yet, blind to our sickness.

According to recent estimates in medical journals, including the April 1999 *Effective Clinical Practice,* three-fourths of the American population has a diagnosable chronic disease. We suffer from many health problems, and most of us take medications to deal with these problems. A 1997 national survey sponsored by *Parade* magazine found that about two-thirds of us regularly take prescription or over-the-counter drugs. This survey also reported that about two-thirds of Americans believe themselves to be in "good" or "excellent" health. My question to you is this: How is it possible to be in good health if you are taking medications and experiencing symptoms of sickness?

Even when statistical evidence is presented, many people fail to recognize their own sickness on a personal level. For example, most people with allergies don't think of themselves as having a chronic disease. Did you know that chronic allergic reactions tax the body and the immune system, making one much more susceptible to infections and other diseases? Allergies are a serious immune dysfunction disease, not just a benign inconvenience. Every allergic reaction does long-term damage to the body; allergies reduce overall quality of life and ultimately reduce longevity. Healthy people do not have allergies.

We think we're healthy, but we're not. At a seminar I was leading, a man stood up and talked about how he jogged every day and how healthy he was. A few pointed questions later, it was revealed that this man had diabetes—the seventh-leading cause of death in America! Some groups assert that we are now healthier and living longer, but that claim seems like propaganda to me. The incidence of virtually every chronic disease continues to increase, and the health of the American people is in a long-term downtrend. In 1996, the *Journal of the American Medical Association* documented that 25 percent of Americans under age eighteen had at least one chronic disease. The disease rate increases to 45 percent between ages forty-five and sixty-five, and to 88 percent over age sixty-five.

Take diabetes, for example. In August 2000, the Centers for Disease Control and Prevention (CDC) announced its most recent statistics on the increases in rates of diabetes. In 1980, 2 percent of newly diagnosed cases of adult-onset diabetes were in people under age nineteen. In 2000, that number was approaching a staggering 50 percent. Separately, in just eight years from 1990 to 1998, diabetes jumped 33 percent nationally and went up a whopping 70 percent among people ages thirty to thirty-nine. According to Dr. Frank Vinicor, the director of the CDC, "This kind of an increase in just eight years is almost unheard of." The experts at the CDC cautioned that even these numbers understate the problem, because about one-third of American diabetics do not realize they have the disease.

Asthma is another example of how fast we are becoming sicker. The CDC reports that the number of Americans with asthma increased 61 percent between 1982 and 1994. Mortality from asthma increased 45 percent between 1985 and 1995. Asthma is now the leading cause of school absenteeism, and the death rate from asthma is increasing at a rate of 6 percent per year.

Obesity is another increasing problem that we must face. Childhood obesity doubled from 1980 to 2000, and most children do not outgrow this problem. Childhood and teenage obesity affects lifelong health with a risk seven times higher for developing clogged arteries later in life. Did you know that more than one in five teenagers are overweight and that almost two of three adults are overweight or obese? Other diseases are increasing, too, including allergies, autoimmune disease, attention deficit disorders, birth defects and chronic fatigue. Cancer is now, after accidents, the leading cause of death for children, and cancer used to be rare in young people!

Would you believe that we have come to expect disease? That we believe in the certainty of sickness more than we believe in the certainty of wellness? That people expect to get sick to such a degree that they hold on to jobs they dislike, just to keep their health benefits? Talk about mixed-up priorities! We are accustomed to disease, and we expect it to occur. When we do get sick, we often feel victimized or helpless, as if struck by a bolt of lightning. We never think that we have done it to ourselves or that we might choose to do otherwise.

Leaving the Good Life

Our lifestyles have changed along with the evolution of what is broadly called "modern civilization." Since the Industrial Revolution, changes have occurred in how we grow our foods, what kinds of food we consume, what we take into our bodies, the lifestyles we live and what we put into the environment. Many of these changes rob us of the nutrients our cells need in order to be healthy and expose us to toxins that interfere with normal cell function. An editorial by Joseph Scherger, M.D., in the January 2000 *Hippocrates* said that "lifestyle factors now loom as the leading cause of premature death."

As I began to discover the incredible health and longevity of certain healthy populations around the world and to look at how these people lived their lives, I began to understand the potential for health. In contrast to the historically healthy populations I will tell you about (such as the Hunzas in northeastern Pakistan and other groups, such as the Vilcabambans and Cuenca Indians in Ecuador), the average American is not doing well at all. We significantly compromise our health with nutritionally deficient diets, environmental toxins, sedentary lifestyles, chronic stress, bad habits such as smoking and drug use, and lack of positive emotions and meaningful relationships, not to mention the damaging outcomes of symptom management by modern medicine. In terms of deficiency and toxicity (the two causes of disease), here are examples of how lifestyle factors make us sick:

Nutrition Failures
- Fruit and vegetable plants are now grown with artificial fertilizers that produce more food per acre, but these foods are not nearly as rich in nutritional content. Use of artificial fertilizers has led to depletion of minerals in the soil because they do not add minerals to replace those

being lost with each new crop. Soil depletion leads to nutritional deficiency in all of us.

- Since foods are not eaten fresh off of the plant, many must be harvested before they are ripe in order to prevent spoilage during transportation and distribution. This premature harvesting does not allow food to reach its full nutritional maturity, thereby contributing to nutritional deficiency.
- The nutritional content of the food then further deteriorates as the food ages during storage, transportation and distribution.
- Food is often processed, further depleting its nutritional content, in order to make it easier to store and consume. Among these foods are flour, pasta, bread, sugar, and canned and packaged foods.
- Cooked foods are also nutritionally inferior to raw ones, and most of the American diet consists of both processed and cooked foods.

Toxic Assaults

- The farming of large single crops has created new and serious problems of insect infestations, necessitating the use of insecticides. These insecticides, along with the use of herbicides and fungicides, have made food production methods a significant contributor to our toxic environment and food supply.
- The modern processed-food industry adds man-made preservatives, flavors, colors and other toxic chemicals to our foods. No one knows what the combination of all these chemicals is doing to our bodies.
- Energy demands, first for coal and now for gas and oil, are constantly polluting our environment.
- Virtually all of our industrial processes—from printing our daily newspapers to painting our homes and building cars and computers—have led to the introduction of tens

of thousands of man-made chemicals into our environment, all of which put toxic loads into our bodies.

Over the past century or so, dramatic changes in diet and environment have created a society of nutritionally deficient and chemically toxic Americans. Virtually all of the food we can buy in a modern supermarket is nutritionally inferior to the foods our ancestors consumed. The purity of the air and water our ancestors enjoyed no longer exists. But all is not lost. Sources do exist today where we can find quality foods with high nutritional content. We can lower our daily toxic exposure, but first we need to learn where to look and how to take charge. What I found helpful was to study those people who have already shown us the way.

Small populations of people in remote areas around the world have shown us how simply meeting the body's needs along each of the six pathways can result in tremendous energy, stamina and lack of disease until age 120, 130 or even older. I will tell you more about these remarkable people, and I will also tell how the intrusions of "modern civilization" into those populations since the 1970s have robbed them of their stunning health and longevity.

Recognizing Our Potential

While 75 is considered a ripe old age in our modern society, traditionally healthy societies considered 75 more "middle age." People in these societies rarely died before their 90s and commonly lived well into their 100s, reaching 120, 130 and older—free of disease. In March 1961, an article in the *Journal of the American Medical Association* reported on evidence that men in Hunza lived to be 120 and even 140 years old. Hunza men and women over 100 exhibited robust energy, in striking contrast to the epidemic of fatigue in our society. These people lived simply and without doctors or hospitals, without nursing homes. In America today we spend $1.5 trillion a year on health care and tens of billions of dollars studying disease. What is it buying us? Certainly not a long, disease-free life. Here's an idea: Study health instead of disease!

So what is our potential for health? In his 1968 book *Hunza,* J. M. Hoffman, Ph.D., who had spent years studying the people of the remote Hunza Valley in the Himalayas, quoted prominent physicians and scientists, including the presidents of the American Medical Association and the International Association of Gerontology, as saying that humans should live to be 120 to 150 years old. Recent estimates in biology journals project human life expectancy to exceed 135 years. Even the Bible itself prophesizes a long life span: "[Man's] days shall be a hundred and twenty years" (Gen. 6:3). Long life is our birthright. We should live to be at least 120, in vigorous health, maintaining physical and mental acuity.

In the state of California, actuarial calculations show that average life expectancy for females would be 100 if only one certain disease were eliminated—heart disease, which is entirely preventable through diet and lifestyle. Consider how much longer we might live by eliminating two or more diseases. Perhaps we have forgotten that health is our natural state. We blindly accept our average life span of seventy-six years; we accept that we will succumb to chronic and degenerative diseases.

Imagining entire populations who have lived far longer and healthier lives than we do seems inconceivable. People who rarely, if ever, suffered from any disease, including colds, allergies, flu or even fatigue. How were these people able to do that? Their nutrition was of high quality, their toxic exposure was minimal, they enjoyed psychological well-being and they were quite physically active. Their everyday lifestyles, to a large degree, met all the factors necessary to support the six pathways toward health.

Let us learn from these people.

The Remarkable Hunzas

In a remote valley of the Himalayas, in what is now north-eastern Pakistan, live the people of Hunza, who were renowned for their near-perfect health, robust energy and extraordinary longevity. Though they lived under what we would consider primitive conditions, they regularly lived into their hundreds, and often lived to be 120 to 140 years old. Their culture was not plagued with cancer, heart disease, ulcers, diabetes, allergies, kidney and liver disease, arthritis, asthma, hypoglycemia, mental disorders, colds, flu, tooth decay or any of the other diseases so common in our society. Nor did they suffer from depression; several researchers described them as, "the happiest people in the world." The Hunzas had clear minds, high intelligence, excellent memories, and enormous physical strength and stamina.

Many researchers went to Hunza in the early twentieth century—long before many of the advances of modern medicine—to study and write about these phenomenally healthy people. Sir Robert McCarrison, M.D., a prominent British physician, spent seven years living and doing research among the Hunzas, and he first brought the health of the Hunza people to world attention. In November 1921, Dr. McCarrison presented the results of his research at a meeting of the Society for Biological Research held at the University of Pittsburgh. He described the Hunzas as, "a race unsurpassed in perfection of physique and in freedom from diseases in general . . ." He found that chronic diseases, including cancer, were totally unknown. (Cancer was unknown among these extraordinarily long-lived people, yet we are told that cancer is a disease of aging.)

Another researcher, J. I. Rodale, in his book, *The Healthy Hunzas,* reported that, "Colds are non-existent in Hunza." He said it was not unusual to see men walking through snowdrifts in the coldest weather, barechested and barefoot. He observed one Hunza man travel sixty miles in a single day, by foot in mountainous terrain, arriving back as if he had returned from a casual walk. Hunza women did not suffer menstrual pain or any of the other female complaints of our society. In Hunza, people typically died of old age in their sleep, without experiencing the chronic suffering that usually precedes death in our own society. The story of the Hunzas shows the potential for human health—how healthy human beings can perform.

As part of their leisure activities, the men of Hunza (from teenage to 120 years old) performed vigorous, physically demanding folk dances. In his book *Hunza,* Hoffman described men in their seventies and eighties gliding through the air with the same grace and ease as those in their teens and twenties. Hoffman wrote: "The stamina of the people is beyond words. In fact men over a hundred years of age were observed going up these mountainsides just as though they were men of fifty. It is my belief that many American men of fifty years of age could not keep up with these Hunza men."

What was it that allowed the Hunzas to achieve this amazing level of health? You probably already know the answer: a combination of a nutritious diet, toxin-free environment, exercise, sleep, sunshine, fresh air and low-stress lifestyle. Given only two causes of disease—deficiency and toxicity—let us examine how the Hunzas kept their cells adequately supplied with nutrients and free of toxins, thus realizing optimal health and longevity. While we cannot replicate their lifestyle, we can see how far our own lifestyles fall short of these goals, and we can begin to understand how to make the kinds of changes that will bring us closer to our potential.

An Optimal Diet and Lifestyle

The Hunza diet was highly nutritious, consisting mainly of vegetarian foods grown in nutrient-rich soil. They irrigated their fields with mineral-rich water and composted all of their organic matter (leaves, straw, manure, etc.), to produce soils of the highest quality. Contrast their mineral-rich soils to U.S. soils which are depleted due to modern chemical farming. It doesn't take a degree in agricultural science to know that if minerals are not in the soil, they do not get into the plant, and then they don't get into you. In addition to fresh vegetables and fruits, the Hunzas ate whole grains that were exceptionally high in nutrients as opposed to the refined sugars and nutrient-depleted white flour that's so prevalent in our diet. Only about 10 percent of the Hunza's calories came from fat, as opposed to about 37 percent in the American diet. Eighty percent of their foods were eaten fresh and raw. In addition to being high in nutrition, their diet was low in toxins, meaning that their foods didn't contain any cancer-causing compounds that come from exposures to pesticides, herbicides, fungicides and other agricultural chemicals. Along with getting plenty of exercise by working the land and walking everywhere, the Hunzas also got adequate sleep. Since there was no artificial lighting in their village, they went to bed when it got dark and they woke up at daybreak, regardless of the time of the year.

So what are we to take from the Hunza's habits? Should we quit our sedentary jobs and take up organic farming? Should we shun all supermarket foods and hide our head under the covers at sunset? While these options are surely not realistic, you can make some practical and positive changes in your lifestyle and this book will show you how. While you don't have to avoid supermarkets altogether, you can learn how to avoid filling your cart with the most toxic foods in the grocery aisles (some of which you might wrongly assume are "healthy" for you!) and paying good money for food that is actually killing you. You can learn how to prepare your foods in ways that don't rob them of their nutrients and how to avoid cooking your foods by methods that compromise your health. You can become aware of what toxic chemicals are lurking in your environment in everyday products and choose healthy alternatives instead. You can see how making a few simple changes in your sleeping habits will restore your body's natural rhythms and allow your body ample time to rejuvenate. You can make informed decisions about which medical treatments you need, and which are actually hurting your health. So, you see, you don't have to move to the Andes Mountains to find health; you can live a long and healthy life in your own town.

And what, you may wonder, would happen to these mighty Hunzas if they lived in your town—with a fast food restaurant on every corner? The results shouldn't surprise you. The Hunzas were geographically isolated from the outside world. The one treacherous road into the Hunza Valley was closed nine months of the year because of the weather, and the road was not all that inviting during the remaining three months. This isolation allowed the Hunzas to live in their traditional, customary, and close-knit familial and social groups, almost up until the present day. Had the Hunza Valley been more accessible, modern culture would have intruded and damaged the health of this population sooner than it did, and we would have lost our opportunity to learn from them. Eventually, modern foods were introduced into the Hunzas' lives when the first all-weather road was built through the mountain passes and into their valley in the 1970s, making this area more accessible to "civilization." "Civilized foods," such as white sugar, white flour, white rice, cola drinks, coffee, processed oils and alcohol were introduced. Fresh, homegrown, whole foods were replaced with the processed and toxic foods that make up much of the diet we eat today. This exposure to modern culture had tremendously detrimental health effects on the Hunza population.

What is especially notable is how rapidly a modern diet will cause health to decline. Researchers have noted that health begins to deteriorate within six months of introducing modern diets into populations previously eating only their traditional foods. The Hunzas were an incredibly healthy population just a few decades ago. Today, they face increasing levels of chronic disease—just like the rest of the "civilized" world. However, because of their prior isolation, the Hunzas provided a perfect control group—an ideal people for the study and measurement of the potential for human health.

If the Hunzas had been the only extraordinarily healthy people in the world, we might dismiss their health as an aberration. However, numerous other examples of long-lived and healthy populations are available, including people living in mountainous areas of Bulgaria and Hungary, the island of Crete, the lake district of Titicaca in Peru, the Vilcabamba Valley in Ecuador, and the Caucasus region of Russia. They all have a similar story. They eat high-quality, nutritious foods. They get a lot of exercise and plenty of fresh air, sleep and sunshine. They live a life of low stress in communities that emphasize family and human relationships. As a result, they enjoy a level of health and quality of life that we can barely imagine.

Unsanitary Conditions, but Healthy People

In another region of Ecuador, we find another story of superior resiliency and longevity: the Indians of the mountainous region of Cuenca. In his book, *How to Survive Modern Technology,* Charles McGee, M.D., reports experiences he had as a Project Hope physician in this region, starting in 1965. McGee had awesome tales to tell about the resilience of these people, who ate excellent diets and lived low-stress lifestyles. Otherwise, however, their living conditions were what we would consider primitive. These Indians usually walked around barefoot and lived in one-room, dirt-floored houses that had no glass in the windows. They had extremely poor sanitary conditions, no running water, no toilet facilities, and their animals wandered haphazardly in and out of their living spaces. As a result of these filthy conditions and a contaminated water supply, infant mortality was very high from bacterial and parasitic infections. (Infants are more susceptible to infections because their immune systems are not yet fully developed.) Examinations of the local children showed that 95 percent had intestinal parasites.

Given the above, one would certainly expect these Indians to be sickly and weak. To the contrary, McGee found them to have perfect teeth, extremely high resistance to infections and amazing resistance to physical trauma resulting from accidents. He described incidents where he treated a man with a ruptured bladder (from a bus accident) and a woman with a ruptured uterus (from childbirth). McGee said that, considering the severity of the damage and the quality of the medical facilities, neither of these people "should have" survived. These people not only survived, they walked home to their mountain villages after treatment at McGee's hospital. Yes, by our standards, they should not have survived; however, our standards are substandard.

Our assumptions about the capabilities of the human body are significantly underestimated. The good nutrition of these people contributed to their cellular health, which allowed them to recover from severe injuries that would have probably killed the typical American. Likewise, absent in these Indians were the typical American diseases, such as heart disease, cancer, diabetes, allergies, asthma, senility and mental illness. Also compelling is that in one year of doing surgery, under very basic and unsanitary conditions, McGee observed only one postoperative infection; in modern, technologically advanced hospitals, infections are bewilderingly rampant. In fact, many people in our society are afraid of hospitals for this exact reason. The resistance to disease of these Indians, under exceptionally challenging conditions, was truly amazing.

Germs and parasites are everywhere, and we have been living with them for millennia. Despite the presence of intestinal parasites in most of the Cuenca, few of them ever became sick from them. Only since the germ theory, and the discovery of microscopic organisms, has medicine focused so obsessively on isolating and killing germs. Medicine has developed few or no protocols for promoting basic human health and immunity, yet promoting health is the only thing that consistently works, as we can see from these healthy populations. The Cuenca had virtually none of the diseases that are so common among us. Why? Because they were fundamentally healthy—that is, they had healthy cells.

McGee contrasted their superior health to the poor health of the population of a nearby city, where toxic junk foods like sugar, white flour, soda pop and white rice had been available for several years. In this city, not surprisingly, heart attacks, diabetes and other chronic diseases had begun to appear.

Modern "Progress"— Toward Deterioration

Having seen how healthy people are capable of performing, living long lives free of disease and enjoying boundless energy, why, with all of our technology, are we doing so poorly by comparison? The many changes we have made in modern society have taken us away from the factors that enhance health and created new conditions that damage health. Never before, in all of human history, have so many health-related factors changed so rapidly and so completely. The basic nutritional, environmental and behavioral dimensions of our society have been severely and rapidly altered. Since the Industrial Revolution, and especially during the past century, humanity has:

• Completely changed its diet.
• Created a new environment.
• Developed new patterns of behavior and lifestyle.

Granted, in this millennium, most of us simply cannot grow

our own food and harvest it when ripe, walk to our destina-
tions, or totally avoid the stresses of modern industrial society.
However, in recognizing what contributed to the health of traditionally healthy people, combined with an understanding of
the significant changes we have made to our own environments and lifestyles, we can begin to see how we must compensate. We need to learn how to create healthy habits for
living within our modern ways of life.

Our way of life is completely different from the lives of
even a century ago. From a personal standpoint, these
changes have been made too slowly for us to notice, but
from an evolutionary standpoint, they have come rapidly—
much too rapidly for healthy adaptation by our bodies and
minds.

The Web of Life

Choosing health would be easy if only one factor were
involved. However, no one factor determines our health.
Rather, our state of health is the end result of countless
biological and behavioral interrelationships called the "web of
life." Unwittingly, we have been busy pulling this web apart,
through the fundamental changes we have made in our diet,
our environment and our behavior. Everything relates to
everything else; making a change in one part of the web
affects the rest of it.

We are learning that life support systems are more interde-
pendent and delicately balanced than we ever realized. No one
fully understands how it all works. The web is as big and complex as the planet itself, and as some scientists suggest, as big
as the universe. But the fact that we do not understand it thoroughly certainly should not prevent us from using what we do
know for protecting and supporting our health right now.

Acting on our knowledge of the factors described in the
chapters about the six pathways can take us beyond "health"

as we have come to accept it. We have seen traditionally healthy people such as the Hunzas achieve a potential for human health that is truly awesome, but to achieve a high level of health in our society requires knowledge, commitment and a willingness to try new things. It can be done. While none of us can or probably want to revert to living a primitive lifestyle, we can, with a few changes in diet and lifestyle, improve our health and quality of life.

3

THE NEW THEORY OF HEALTH AND DISEASE

One Disease

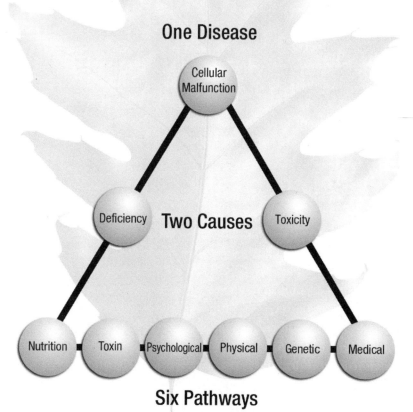

Cellular Malfunction

Deficiency **Two Causes** Toxicity

Nutrition   Toxin   Psychological   Physical   Genetic   Medical

Six Pathways

"The most basic weapons in the fight against disease are the most ignored by modern medicine: the numerous nutrients the cells of our bodies need. *If our body cells are ailing—as they must be in disease—the chances are excellent that it is because they are being inadequately provisioned."*

Roger J. Williams, Ph.D.
Nutrition Against Disease

odern medicine believes that thousands of diseases exist, each with different causes and treatments. This belief has led to a system of medicine so complex and baffling that physicians resort to protocols that merely suppress symptoms. By suppressing symptoms rather than addressing causes, diseases remain chronic. In this chapter, you will learn a new approach. This new theory of health and disease is a model that recognizes not thousands of diseases but only one disease, along with only two causes of disease. This simple model of disease is so powerful that it can enable you to go beyond health as you have experienced it and never be sick again.

One Disease—Two Causes—
Six Pathways

A real understanding of the relationship between health and disease cannot be achieved through knowledge of germs, inherited genes, medicines, surgery, or any of the many "diseases" that make people sick. Keeping up with these subjects is complex and doesn't really help people to take care of themselves. What we need right now are solutions for good health. The time is ripe to simplify: Understand what your cells need, how they work and what causes them to malfunction. Your cells are what make your life possible.

There is only one disease: **malfunctioning cells.**

When cells malfunction, the body is no longer able to maintain homeostasis (balance) by regulating and repairing itself. This is the essence of disease, no matter what you call it or how it happens. Because only one disease exists, all we need to do is prevent the causes of that one disease.

There are only two causes of disease:
deficiency *and* **toxicity.**

All you have to do for health is to give your cells what they need and protect them from what they don't need. Cells malfunction only if they suffer from a lack of nutrients (deficiency), toxic damage (toxicity) or a combination of both. Preventing these two causes of disease is made possible by our ability to choose how we live our lives. Health depends on the choices we make. These choices fall into six categories, or pathways.

> **There are six pathways between health and disease:**
> **nutrition, toxin, psychological, physical,**
> **genetic *and* medical.**

The body knows how to take care of itself, provided it has what it needs to do so. Good choices along the six pathways provide for the needs of your body just as sunshine, water and rich soil provide for the needs of a houseplant. These concepts are not complicated; in fact they are incredibly simple. We just become lost along the way sometimes because we don't have a sound theory of health and disease. Well, now we do: one disease, two causes, six pathways. Applying this theory can restore balance to your cells and support your cells' natural ability to self-regulate and repair damage. Along each of the six pathways, I teach you in this book how to prevent the two causes of disease. Using this knowledge, you can restore health and prevent future sickness.

The Need to Simplify

At the time of my illness, despite my scientific education and background, I probably knew as much, or as little, about disease as most people. I thought that disease was something that came from germs and from genetic predisposition. I thought disease was something that happened to the unlucky, the starving, or to those who really abused themselves, such as alcoholics and drug addicts. My physician said that my problems were the result of aging, as opposed to something that I had unknowingly chosen and could choose to reverse.

During my recovery process, I realized that I would have been able to prevent my illness if I had understood the causes of disease. I realized that as long as disease remained something mysterious, complicated and difficult to understand, then only the high priests of medicine—the educated experts we call doctors—would be able to deal with it. What if we could all understand what causes disease? Wouldn't we be empowered to prevent disease? Can we actually do that? Can we distill simple truth from this complex mystery? Throughout man's history, great advancements in science have often come from people who were able to take extraordinarily complex subjects and simplify them. In this chapter we are trying to simplify the concepts of health and disease.

Simplifying Disease

Consider this: Rather than thousands of diseases, there is only one disease. Does this sound ridiculous? Probably, but that is because we are conditioned to think of many different diseases, rather than recognizing what is common to all disease. The most difficult aspect of this theory is that it requires you to look at health and disease in a completely different way. Using the concept of one disease dramatically simplifies how we perceive disease in general.

To simplify disease, we must first have an understanding of what disease is. In order to do that, we need a basic understanding of *cells*. Every plant and animal on earth is made of cells—the smallest unit of life. Fossil records show that the earliest forms of life were single-celled organisms. Likewise, each human being started as one cell—a single cell encoded with all of the information needed to develop into the vastly complex, multitrillion-celled organisms that we are today.

Each of us is made of about seventy-five trillion cells. Not all of these cells are the same. Humans have over 200 different types of cells (nerve cells, blood cells, muscle cells, bone cells, etc.), forming many different types of tissues that enable us to eat, breathe, feel, move, think and reproduce. Together, cells combine to form the building blocks of biological structure and function. All of these cells communicate with each other and rely on these communications in order to keep us alive and well.

Healthy cells make healthy tissues, which are highly resistant to disease and physical injury. Unhealthy cells create unhealthy tissues, which are quite susceptible to both disease and injury.

What Is Disease?

Each cell must perform specific tasks in order to collaborate effectively with other cells in the body. If all of your cells are healthy, these tasks are well executed and the body functions at optimal levels. *If all of your cells are healthy, you cannot be sick.* If, for any reason, a cell starts to malfunction, it is less able to perform its assigned tasks, which is where problems can begin. When such malfunction occurs in a large enough number of cells to impair the body's ability to self-repair and self-regulate, disease occurs.

The scientific term for a cell that is malfunctioning is *cytopathy* (*cyto* referring to cell, and *pathy* to sickness or disease). As fantastically complex as we humans are, the fundamental concept of disease is simple. *Disease is the result of a large number of malfunctioning cells (widespread cytopathy).* This definition is not fancy or eloquent; it may even seem absurdly simple. However, it is a profound, precise and irrefutable definition of disease. This definition is so simple that no one—scientist, physician or layperson—can deny it. This definition provides the unifying theory of health and disease that the modern medical establishment lacks, which is the reason that modern medicine is unable to address the current epidemic of chronic disease.

Perhaps you are thinking, "But wait! Disease is much more complex than that! What about genetic predisposition? What about bacterial and viral infection? What about cancer? What about AIDS? What about . . . ?" True, many factors may conspire in contributing to the malfunction of our cells and the many different ways in which they can malfunction. In the end, though, cellular malfunction creates the measurable abnormalities that we call disease. Therefore, no matter which cells malfunction, or why they malfunction, *the malfunction is the one disease.*

A person cannot be sick unless a large number of cells are malfunctioning. The first steps on the path to disease are taken when, for whatever reason, a single cell begins to malfunction, and then another cell and another. When the number grows large enough, we may begin to notice. We may "feel sick" along the way, perhaps experiencing a pain here, a discomfort there or a lack of energy. By the time your health has deteriorated into a diagnosable chronic disease, no cell may be left in your body that is still functioning optimally. I am astounded when people describe their health problems and then claim that, "other than this," they are in excellent health!

Unfortunately, modern medicine finds itself mired in complexity, confronted with numerous diseases, diagnoses and treatments. Lost in the midst of thousands of different diseases (each supposedly with its own unique causes), physicians are unable to effectively diminish disease in our society. A simpler and more effective solution is to focus on the process—the one disease—and to ask what causes it. When you understand disease as a process, rather than a "thing" to be cut out or suppressed, then you see why surgery and drugs, virtually the only tools of the physician, are limited in what they can do.

The Two Causes of Disease

Cellular malfunction is the essence of disease. But why does it happen? Cells can malfunction in a multitude of ways, and the biochemistry of these malfunctions can be exceedingly complex. All malfunctions can be reduced to two causes: *deficiency* and *toxicity*. *Deficiency* means that cells are lacking something that they need in order to function the way they are designed to function. *Toxicity* means that cells are poisoned by something that inhibits proper function. Either one of these factors—and usually a combination of both—can and will cause disease.

One of the great scientific minds of the twentieth century, biochemist Dr. Roger Williams, wrote, "Body cells in general die for two reasons: First, because they do not get everything they need; second, because they get poisoned by something they decidedly do not need." Humans can live long and healthy lives if we do two things right: provide our cells with all of the nutrients they need and protect our cells from toxins. To the extent that we can accomplish these tasks well, we can significantly extend the length and the quality of our lives. In the real world, these two tasks are never accomplished perfectly. As a result, cells suffer, we age, the quality of life is diminished and we die. The variable in this sequence is how fast we allow this to happen.

What about other causes of disease, such as genetic inheritance and infections by microorganisms? Yes, genes and germs trigger cellular malfunction, but they do so by causing deficiencies or toxicities, which are always the common denominators of disease. Eliminate these factors and you eliminate disease. For example, consider diseases with a genetic basis, such as ALD (adrenoleukodystrophy), the genetic disease featured in the movie *Lorenzo's Oil*. People with ALD develop abnormally high levels of very long-chain fatty acids, which are molecules that are natural to the body. These fatty acids can build up to levels that are toxic to cells. This *toxicity* is the result of a genetically caused *deficiency* of special protein molecules that keep these fatty acid levels within normal limits. Lorenzo's parents compensated for the genetic deficiency by supplementing their son's diet with a combination of oils that helped to lower the level of the offending fatty acids, thereby reducing the toxic effect on his body. What caused Lorenzo's disease? Was it genetics? Yes, but for his disease to manifest, his cells had to be deficient and toxic. *Deficiency and toxicity are always the common denominators of all disease.* The same is true of infections from microorganisms. Anthrax, for example, makes us sick and kills by producing toxins. Without deficiency and toxicity causing cells to malfunction, there is no disease.

What about stress? Hasn't that been proven to cause disease? True, stress is a major factor that contributes to disease. Chronic stress results in an excessive buildup of natural chemicals in the body, which at higher levels become toxic. In addition, stress depletes the body of certain nutrients, resulting in deficiency. Stress is a contributor to disease, but only by expressing itself through the common denominators of all disease: deficiency and toxicity.

Deficiency and toxicity, regardless of their cause, increasingly compromise the functioning of cells, making a person steadily more vulnerable to developing a diagnosable disease. By the time you contract a diagnosable disease (whether we're talking about the common cold, allergies, cancer or heart disease), you have probably been "sick" for a long time. You have suffered enough cellular damage from deficiency and toxicity that cells throughout your body are malfunctioning. You *are* sick long before you *get* sick. By the time symptoms are produced, cellular malfunction has become widespread, cell-to-cell communications have been disrupted and the systemic manifestations are the symptoms. Remember that disease does not just randomly happen, like a meteorite falling out of the sky. Health, not disease, is the natural state of human existence, but forgetting this point is easy when we see all the disease around us.

Symptoms Versus the One Disease

Our society's current understanding of disease is based on the concept of *symptomology*. *Symptomology* is about focusing on, identifying and categorizing symptoms—in other words, the effects produced by disease. In this manner, doctors supposedly can differentiate one disease from another. Because the entirety of modern medicine and everything we have ever learned about disease is based on symptomology, the concept of only one disease may seem unacceptably simplistic. Actually the symptomology concept is the flawed one.

Symptomology is based on a fundamental misconception, one held by virtually all medical establishments in Western society. The misconception is that thousands of different diseases exist, each with different symptoms, causes and treatments. This misconception stems from the many different ways that cells can malfunction, and therefore the thousands of different symptoms that can be produced. The modern medical treatment of almost all disease focuses on the management of these symptoms (the effects of disease), rather than eliminating the causes, which are deficiency and toxicity. People are told to take insulin to manage their blood sugar rather than eliminating their diabetes, or to take diuretics to treat their hypertension rather than normalizing their blood pressure. They are told to have a bypass operation rather than reversing their heart disease or to undergo chemotherapy rather than healing their cancer.

Diagnosis by symptoms is the process by which modern medicine gives each collection of symptoms a particular name. Medicine views symptoms as enemies, and physicians are trained to eliminate them, even if that means aggressively assaulting the body with dangerous toxins, radiation or invasive surgery. Symptomology leads the medical profession to look at symptoms individually, organize them into thousands of categories, label them as different diseases and then prescribe a currently accepted protocol to suppress those symptoms. This approach adds needless complexity, creates massive confusion and results in an inability to deal with disease in a meaningful way.

In truth, each collection of symptoms—each specific "disease"—is just a different expression of malfunctioning cells. However, with all of our different types of cells, and all of the different ways in which each cell can malfunction, the number of possible combinations of symptoms becomes vast. In other words, when cells malfunction, we may feel sick in many different ways.

Cells that are malfunctioning because of a vitamin C deficiency exhibit different symptoms than those malfunctioning because of a zinc deficiency. Cells malfunctioning because of lead toxicity exhibit different symptoms from those malfunctioning because of mercury toxicity. Various combinations of deficiencies and toxicities produce a myriad of complex symptoms (thousands of "diseases"), but the symptoms are not relevant. To solve any problem, you have to address the causes, not the symptoms.

Modern medicine, by placing the focus on symptoms, has yet to develop any theory regarding the relationship between health and disease. Medicine looks at these as if they are two different states, while health and disease are really different sides of the same coin in a constantly shifting continuum. Lacking a practical theory, physicians have no framework in which to understand health or how to help patients achieve it, like being lost in a vast jungle without a map or compass. Narrowly trained, our physicians are taught the art of surgery and the administration of drugs as tools to manage symptoms. If the only tool you have is a hammer, so the saying goes, then every problem looks like a nail. If you go to a conventionally trained physician, then medicine's "hammers"—surgery and drugs—are what you receive. Unfortunately, these tools are designed to manage and suppress symptoms, not to cure disease.

For a more meaningful understanding of disease (cellular malfunction), we must consider the health of our cells. Remember that noticeable health problems begin when a large number of cells malfunction. As this happens, important cellular chemicals are not produced, cell-to-cell communications become garbled and the body ceases to regulate itself properly. Our tissues suffer and noticeable symptoms appear, e.g., allergies, fatigue, aches and pains, colds, flu, depression, anxiety, cancer or any of thousands of other complaints.

Categorizing and suppressing the symptoms of malfunctioning cells does not fix the problem. This approach cannot explain why the problem occurred in the first place, cannot prevent the problem from happening again and cannot prevent it from appearing elsewhere in the body. The only "cure" is to restore our cells and tissues to health.

What Is Health?

Everybody thinks they know what health is, but people asked to define it give you many different answers. In order to define health, perhaps we first should provide the definition of health used in modern medicine: "Health is the absence of disease." This medical school lesson is not a very good definition. For medicine to recognize disease, it must be diagnosable. You are not sick until the day the physician can diagnose something. The absence of diagnosable disease is not a good working definition of health. *Modern medicine has no way of recognizing or diagnosing disease when your health is in its initial decline.* When I was sick and already experiencing disturbing symptoms, my physician pronounced me in excellent health. He had never been taught how to notice and measure my already extensive decline in health. We are considered sick only after the problem has become serious enough to produce symptoms that fit neatly into one of medicine's disease categories. This way of looking at health is not helpful, productive or self-empowering. Health is much more than the absence of a diagnosable disease.

When your cells are functioning as they should, you have ample adaptive capacity to thrive in our constantly changing environment without ill effects. With properly functioning cells, you have strong resilience to various kinds of stress— physical, chemical, biological and emotional. You have the ability to make daily repairs to your cells, the ability to build healthy new ones, and the ability to efficiently remove pathogenic microorganisms and toxins from your body. You become an optimally balanced organism, with integrated mental and physical equilibrium. Perhaps most important is that achieving good cellular health gives our society the ability to produce healthy offspring.

While the above descriptions explain the practical effects of health, they still do not offer a single, concrete definition of health. In order to clearly define health, as a concept concrete enough to be understood and discussed, let us work with the following definition:

Health is the state wherein all cells are functioning optimally.

Never are all of our cells functioning perfectly, so the challenge is to keep cellular malfunction to a minimum. Even in healthy people, cells are constantly being damaged, dying and being replaced. Our bodies produce more than 10 million new cells every second, as we constantly rebuild our tissues. How healthy are each of these new cells? If we replace sick cells with sick cells, we will never recover. As cells die off are we replacing them with healthy cells or sick cells?

Who Succumbs to Disease?

Only sick people become sick. Once you start to compromise health, a cascade of events follow. Once a critical number of cells begin to malfunction, internal communications and self-regulation systems become debilitated and destabilized. As the number of compromised cells increases, the effects are compounded. Before anyone can exhibit noticeable signs of disease, normal cell function has to be compromised significantly throughout the body. Vulnerability to infections, for example, is created by widespread cellular malfunction. An infection indicates that cellular malfunction already has weakened the immune system. Having a cold or the flu is an alarm screaming at you that all is not well, because healthy people resist infections in the first place. Few of us pay attention to these alarms. We think that having a cold or the flu is normal, and that once the symptoms are gone we are well again. Not so.

The level of your health and immunity determines whether or not the presence of a microorganism results in an infection. *You are already sick before you come down with an infection.* Otherwise everybody who is exposed to a given "bug" would become sick, which is not the case. Contrary to the common notion that we "catch" diseases, people become sick only after their cellular health is already compromised. Disease (cellular malfunction) comes first; active infections and chronic problems follow.

The skeptic says, "But he was born with asthma and suffered from it as an infant." "She was in the best of health, took great care of herself, and then suddenly got breast cancer." Although we hear these kinds of statements frequently, the notion is flawed that a person is a powerless victim of disease. This way of looking at events comes from living in a society that does not have an accurate understanding of disease, or of what is required to create and maintain health.

Think of the historically healthy societies, such as the Hunzas. These people implicitly understood what they needed to maintain their health. They lived far longer than we do, without the chronic degenerative diseases from which we suffer. The principles of good health were built into their beliefs and lifestyles. The key lesson to be learned from these people is this:

Healthy people do not get sick.

Most of us have not learned to think this way. We grow up in a society where almost everyone has a chronic disease. We have been taught, through experience, that disease is a "normal" part of the aging process. Diseased people are typically seen as the helpless victims of an inevitable and "natural" process. Especially when the symptoms of disease develop suddenly, people feel surprised and victimized. Yet, the two causes were there all the time, gradually wearing down cellular competence and creating an opportunity for disease to "strike."

As part of the body's normal maintenance and repair process, old cells are constantly being replaced with new ones. If new cells are not built with proper raw materials, they will be unhealthy and weak. Such cells are unable to perform their normal tasks, including routine repairs, and will be vulnerable to sickness and injury. Ultimately, the body's self-regulation systems will break down. Because of the poor diets and the toxic environment in our society, cells are often deficient and toxic when first created, becoming progressively more so over time. This situation is precarious, with a large number of cells either malfunctioning or functioning at a borderline level. Similar to walking a tightrope, falling off is easy. Any number of stressful factors can affect a person adversely who is already deficient and toxic, be it a stressful event, a pathogenic organism, a night out on the town, a physical injury or even a lengthy airplane flight. Almost any challenge to a compromised system can be the straw that breaks the overburdened camel's back.

Though painful to acknowledge, disease sufferers invariably (if unknowingly) have made poor choices leading to illness. In the case of sick children, the parents have made the poor choices.

We are not taught that we have the ability to and, in fact, need to consistently make meaningful choices about our health. Instead, when we become sick we look to something outside of ourselves to explain our "misfortune." We look for some obvious circumstance that can explain why we are sick. Do these excuses sound familiar? "I walked outside in the cold air and . . ." or "So and so was coughing and sneezing near me at work and . . ." or "Everybody at little Ricky's school is sick, it's no wonder that . . ." or "Obesity runs in my family . . ." We are accustomed to ill health as something that mysteriously lands on us. We fail to see our own role regarding its development. When invited to consider illness as the result of our poor choices, usually we reject such a notion. *By placing the blame for sickness on excuses, we relieve ourselves of responsibility.*

However, accepting responsibility for our health can be enormously empowering. The overall competence of cells— determined by relative levels of deficiency and toxicity—are the sole determinants of health. Learn how to embrace health and avoid illness by educating yourself in how to make healthful choices that lower your levels of deficiency and toxicity and promote your cellular health.

In Which Direction Is Your Health Moving?

Some of the time we are sick, and most of the time we are well. This variability in our individual health is almost exclusively the result of the choices we make. In this fluctuation, sickness is not the absolute opposite of health. Health and sickness are not fixed concepts and they cannot be defined in black-and-white terms. Instead, consider your health as a constantly changing continuum. Consider the balance between sickness and health as a scale, with optimal health at one end, and death at the other. Somewhere in between is a diagnosable disease. As life progresses, your position on the scale shifts, moving back and forth all the time. At any time, it is worthwhile to ask: Where am I on this scale? In which direction on this scale am I moving?

The Health and Performance Scale shown on the next page is simple but effective, serving to illustrate the relationship between sickness and health. In considering this diagram, remember our definitions of health and disease. Optimal health (on the far right) is that theoretical state in which every cell is functioning optimally and you are absolutely as healthy as your genetic capacity allows. This condition is called *homeostasis*—when the body is perfectly in balance and continually is fine-tuning itself to maintain that balance. Very few Americans are at this end of the scale, but we should strive toward this goal. Between optimal health and death is diagnosable disease. In this state, cellular malfunction is occurring on such a large scale that the symptoms of a medically defined disease are produced. On the far left of the scale is death—where all cells have ceased to function.

The Health and Performance Scale

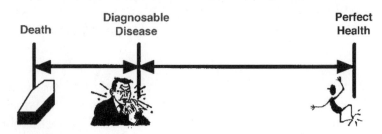

©2002 *Beyond Health*

Tragically, more than three out of four Americans have medically significant cellular malfunction—a diagnosable disease of some kind. The overwhelming majority of us are somewhere between diagnosable disease and death!

Think about your personal health equation, your position on this Health and Performance Scale. Do you have a diagnosable disease? If so, you are located between disease and death. Even without having a diagnosable disease, your health may be far from optimal. Fortunately, your position on this continuum is not static; it can change depending on your choices.

No matter your age or your current state of health, you have the power to change the direction in which you are going and how rapidly you move on the Health and Performance Scale. I learned this firsthand, in making powerful life-saving choices, after it was declared a medical certainty that I would die. I learned it again years later, after witnessing the illness and extraordinary recovery of an elderly woman.

A family called me to ask for help with their bedridden and senile mother. This woman was ninety-four years old and unable to get out of bed; sometimes she recognized her family and knew where she was, at other times she did not. Her children loved her very much and did not want to place her in a nursing home, yet the burden of her care had become too much for them. With nowhere else to turn, they asked if there was anything I could recommend. My reply was, "Probably not." Given the woman's debilitated condition, I assumed that her health had deteriorated beyond repair. At a certain point, enough cellular machinery has been damaged that sufficient repairs can no longer be made. Though I was pessimistic about the likelihood of any improvement, the family asked for my advice anyway. In retrospect, I found out that I still had a lot to learn about the capacity of the human body to heal itself.

I started out by recommending some specific vitamin supplements to help supply certain key nutrients to her cells. When I asked what she was eating, the first item they mentioned was milk. After years of study, I had come to realize that cow's milk is not an appropriate food for any human being. For someone in her condition, cow's milk was almost certainly putting a toxic load on her already struggling body. I recommended that they stop feeding her milk. As I hung up the phone, I doubted that these suggestions would have much of an impact or that I would ever hear from them again. Two weeks later the phone rang with gleeful reports of her "miraculous" improvement. She was getting out of bed, going to the bathroom and getting dressed—all by herself. She was walking around the house and having rational conversations with her family. A miracle? No, just a movement of her health equation in the right direction. By addressing her cellular deficiency and toxicity, this woman's body began once again to repair and regulate itself. Indeed, I have learned that almost anyone can alter his or her health equation in a positive direction.

Sickness never happens without a cause. The cause is usually our own ignorance of or disregard for our personal health equations. So how can you avoid getting sick? Simple. Make the kind of health-conscious life choices that optimize your personal health equation. We live in a fast-paced society that has created an environment and adopted diets, lifestyles and behaviors that do not support human health. If we want to be healthy, we have to make choices that significantly deviate from the diet and lifestyle of the average American. Eating a "normal" diet and living a "normal" life are virtually guaranteed to make you sick. To prevent this from happening, you must be proactive. As Joseph D. Beasley, M.D., said in *The Kellogg Report,* "In the long run, individuals cannot be better than their biology—as affected by their nutrition, ecology, and lifestyle."

The key to never having to be sick again is the ability to choose between the things that are healthy and the things that are not. This sounds simple, but accurate information about what is healthy is hard to come by. Next, let's look at a definition and an overview of each of the six pathways between health and disease and explain how knowledge of them can lead to better decisions about health.

The Six Pathways Between Health and Disease

Having read this far, has your perspective on health and disease changed? Are you becoming accustomed to the theory of one disease and two causes? You have learned that if your cells malfunction to the degree that they interfere with your body's ability to balance and regulate itself, you are diseased. Whether you are suffering from the flu, cancer, diabetes, depression or something else, cellular malfunction is always the essence of the problem.

The tool that I developed to help myself make better choices is the six pathways. As demonstrated, your personal health equation is always in flux; depending on the choices you make, you will move either in the direction of optimal health or in the direction of disease and death. This movement occurs along the six pathways. These six pathways are like six different roads; each spans the distance between health and disease. Depending on the choices made along each pathway, you are moving toward one or the other. The six pathways concept provides a framework through which informed, logical, health-enhancing choices can be made.

The pathways are:

- Nutrition
- Toxin
- Psychological
- Physical
- Genetic
- Medical

A holistic approach to health requires attention to all of these pathways. Consistent movement in the wrong direction along any of them can lead to cellular malfunction, breakdown of self-regulation and diagnosable disease. Continuous movement in the right direction leads to optimal health and performance.

By learning about the six pathways, you can have a clear understanding of the different ways that health can be influenced. You will be empowered to mitigate the negative effects of modern living, thus taking charge of your personal health.

Pathway Number One: Nutrition

What is America's leading cause of disease? *Malnutrition.* We think of ourselves as so well fed that the idea that we are suffering from malnutrition is difficult for most Americans to grasp. When we hear the word "malnourished," we recall television images of starving children. Although Americans are rarely undernourished to this extent, we are malnourished, and in fact it is our leading cause of disease. The typical diet, what most Americans eat, simply does not supply sufficient nutrients. No wonder that we suffer from the one disease in its various forms.

The nutrition pathway is about the relationship between the nutritional content of your diet and your health. Obtaining proper nutritional intake on a daily basis is important because nutrients act as a team. A shortage of even one nutrient will decrease the effectiveness of all the others. Nutritional status affects our entire being, including moods and emotions, the ability to learn and remember, physical performance and resistance to disease. Cells and tissues thrive when provided with an environment rich in nutrients such as water, oxygen, vitamins, minerals, proteins, carbohydrates and essential fatty acids, while deficiency causes disease and shortens life.

To some degree, almost all Americans are overfed but undernourished. Virtually everything that we eat today, unless we make special choices, is nutritionally inferior to the foods that our ancestors were eating as recently as a few generations ago. Not only have we fundamentally changed what we eat; we have changed how our food is grown, processed, transported, stored, treated and prepared. These changes cause our foods to be nutritionally deficient—the primary cause of our modern epidemic of chronic disease. In addition, our crops usually retain toxic residues from pesticides and other agricultural chemicals, and some are even ripened with artificial chemicals. Both nutritionally deficient and chemically toxic, our modern food supply promotes disease.

Pathway Number Two: Toxin

Toxins interfere with normal cell function, thereby causing malfunctions. Most people know that toxins are dangerous, but what are toxins, and how do toxins damage our cells?

We are exposed to toxins in various ways: in the air we

breathe, the water we drink, the clothes we wear and the food we eat. In our modern world, we are exposed to these environmental toxins all day, every day. Toxins in our environment can impose an undue external burden on us, while poor digestion, lack of exercise, and negative thoughts and emotions can increase our toxic loads internally.

Our bodies do have the ability to detoxify, but our detoxification mechanisms require essential nutrients to function properly. Inadequate nutrition deprives the body of the raw materials necessary to detoxify, so toxic levels build and negatively affect cellular health. In our society, toxic overload is having a bigger effect than it should, because our deficient diets do not supply the nutrients necessary to operate and maintain our detoxification mechanisms. Not only is our toxic load the highest in history, but our ability to process and eliminate these toxins is impaired.

Because we know that excessive toxic exposure causes disease, learning about the toxin pathway can teach us which substances are toxic, how toxic they are, where they are, how they get there and how we can minimize our exposures to them. The toxin pathway provides insight into the toxic aspects of our daily lives—in our food supply, water supply, homes and personal products (including many soaps, shampoos and toothpastes). Fortunately, healthful alternatives are available. Toxic exposure is a fact of life, and the body is designed to deal with it. Our problem is toxic overload, i.e., when the toxic input exceeds our ability to process it. Understanding this pathway can help us to reduce toxic exposure to manageable levels by teaching us to recognize and avoid toxins in our daily lives.

Pathway Number Three: Psychological

The psychological pathway may turn out to be the most important pathway of all. Through study of the psychological pathway, we learn about the significance of thoughts, emotions and behavior, and how these affect our health.

Many people believe that the mind has an enormous effect on the body. This idea, however, is based on the supposition that the mind somehow is separated from the body. In truth, the entire body, including the brain, is the mind. When we understand that the mind and body are one, reports of placebo effects and miraculous healings should not be surprising. In fact, they are part of everyday life.

Our thoughts and emotions trigger a cascade of biochemical reactions that either enhance or damage health. How we react to various life events and how we respond to our thoughts and emotions are choices that can damage or enhance cellular health. What we allow to enter our minds on a daily basis is critical. What we think and feel over a lifetime plays a major role in our health or illness. The significance and impact of the factors associated with this pathway may indeed be more important than all the nutrients and toxins we put into our bodies, perhaps even more important than all the other pathways put together. The psychological pathway explores the subjects relevant to behavioral and psychological factors in health and disease, including meditation, stress, thoughts, emotions and the placebo effect.

Pathway Number Four: Physical

The physical pathway contains recommendations on how to recognize and provide for the body's physical needs. This pathway can be used to enhance physical potential and to minimize physical damage. Just as nutrition and toxic avoidance are important to health, physical maintenance and care are also essential to the health equation.

Most Americans do not get adequate exercise, sleep or sunlight. An indoor, sedentary lifestyle means little or no exercise nor exposure to natural light. Our mental lifestyle, meanwhile, is excessively fast paced, and this, together with a high incidence of sleep deprivation, means that often we are chronically and seriously stressed. Also we are exposed to subtle physical influences, such as electromagnetic fields caused by the wiring in our homes, hairdryers, heaters, electric razors, cell phones and the X rays we receive as part of medical and dental evaluations.

Pathway Number Five: Genetic

Limit genetic damage. Optimize genetic potential. These are the goals we strive toward on the genetic pathway.

The genetic pathway focuses on optimizing the expression of our genes to promote health and limit any damage to the genes. Each human being is genetically unique; inherent strengths and weaknesses are a part of our basic genetic makeup. Genes are the blueprint of life. Our genes, however, rarely have the final say and they are certainly not the primary cause of disease that modern medicine would have us believe. Genes are a potential for expression, and they express themselves in ways commensurate with life's circumstances.

The genetic pathway explores topics such as the genetic causes for disease and the effects of genetically engineered foods. Further, this pathway identifies specific hazards that can potentially cause genetic damage, such as environmental chemicals, prescription drugs and radiation. Most important is the personal resolve of individuals to commit themselves seriously to optimizing health, rather than accepting their so-called genetic predisposition as a fore-doomed fate.

Pathway Number Six: Medical

The medical pathway is perhaps the most surprising and most misunderstood of all the pathways. As we have noted, many people rave about and swear by the near-miraculous feats accomplished by modern medicine. The technology that contemporary medicine has to offer is best used in crisis intervention and trauma care. However, such applications are limited. No doubt that physicians are well-meaning, but a blind trust in them and in the treatments they offer (surgery and drugs) to the exclusion of other considerations can lead to destructive and even lethal consequences.

The medical pathway helps to explain how modern medicine can cause disease. Widespread ignorance and failure to comprehend this fact are reasons that modern medicine harms the health of our population. By studying this pathway we can identify and avoid potentially harmful aspects of medicine, while still reaping the benefits of modern medical technology.

The medical pathway is unique, expressing itself through all of the other pathways and thus, compromising health at many levels. In working to optimize your personal health equation, you need to be aware of the ways in which modern medical "care" actually can damage your health along any of the other pathways. Chapter 10 about the medical pathway describes more specifically medicine's capabilities and its limitations.

A New Theory for a New Millennium

During the last century, modern industrial society has brought fundamental changes to human existence; we are developing and changing the world much faster than our biology can adapt. Today, nutritional intake, toxic exposures and stress levels bear little resemblance to those of even our most recent biological ancestors. Every cell in our bodies is adversely affected by these profound changes, which is why our society has suffered more and more chronic disease. Disease is the catastrophic result of decades of inadequate nutrition, toxic exposures, sedentary lifestyles, familial and social disruptions and a dependence on drugs (prescription, over-the-counter and recreational).

In this chapter, I have attempted to outline the complexity and confusion that surround disease in our society. I offer a new theory of health and disease, a new way to look at these concepts: There is only one disease, cellular malfunction, and only two causes of disease, deficiency and toxicity. Six pathways can lead to health or disease. Our confusion arises because cells malfunction in many different ways. Modern medicine categorizes the symptoms created by these various malfunctions as different diseases, even though they have common causes. Achieving victory over disease requires removing the causes. Eliminate deficiency and toxicity, allow the body to self-repair and self-regulate, and disease will go away.

4

CHOOSING
HEALTHY CELLS

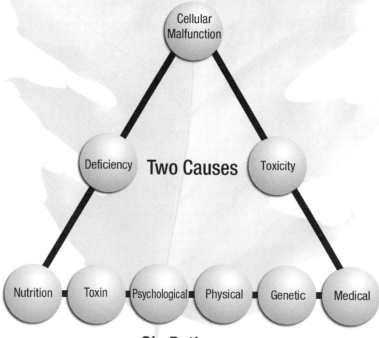

One Disease

Cellular
Malfunction

Deficiency   **Two Causes**   Toxicity

Nutrition   Toxin   Psychological   Physical   Genetic   Medical

Six Pathways

"Cells—in the skin, the muscles, the lungs, the liver, the intestines, the kidneys, the blood vessels, the glands, the heart and, crucially, the nerves and brain—must be well nourished if we are to lead long and healthy lives. Contrarily, if these cells are undernourished, disabilities and diseases of every description will ensue."

Roger J. Williams, Ph.D.
Nutrition Against Disease

L et us take a trip together to the front lines of the daily battle between health and disease: your cells. Cells are the building blocks of your body. They build your tissues, and these tissues make up your systems. Because malfunctioning cells are the one disease, learning to care for cells is fundamental to healthy living. Come with me on a tour of the systems that keep your body healthy or that make you sick. The struggle for life itself occurs within every cell. The vitality of a person can only be as strong as the cells of which they are made.

The basics of caring for your cells are as follows:

- Supply cells with all the raw materials they need.
- Avoid the damaging effects of toxic chemicals.

- Build healthy cell membranes, the cell's first line of defense against disease.
- Learn how to prevent and reverse disease by understanding how cells work and how they malfunction.
- Choices, rather than genetic inheritance, are key.

Lost Along the Way

Before we leave our homes to travel—particularly if our destination is unfamiliar—we usually spend time reading brochures, studying maps, or researching local customs, currency, and, perhaps, health precautions. We rarely give that kind of attention to our own bodies and to our health, yet what could be more important?

Most people expect that their bodies generally take care of themselves, provided they don't smoke, drink to excess, or fall prey to some unstoppable virus or some predetermined genetic disease. Most people believe that as long as they avoid "fattening" foods, they are eating a healthful diet. On all counts, these people are wrong.

One of the most important things you need in order to fight disease and to encourage your own health is knowledge. This chapter teaches you how to prepare and what to pack for a healthy journey through the rest of your life. The small amount of time you will spend reading this chapter will be an investment worth making: It may save your life. Knowledge is power, and you are about to plug into a tremendous energy source.

A cabinet stocked with medicines, a list of doctors to call, and a head filled with commercial endorsements, medical studies and drug warning labels does nothing to give you what you really need: a true understanding of what makes you sick or how to get well. Without that understanding, you can be caught up in a whirlwind of medical procedures and pharmaceuticals that suppress or surgically remove the symptoms of what are labeled as thousands of different diseases. In reality, these drugs and surgeries do not cure disease, and they may actually kill you. Despite the confusion out there about how disease occurs and the different health plans that seek to promote health, real success can only come if you keep your cells working right. This chapter teaches you, simply and clearly, how your body works at its most basic level: your cells.

The Cell

A cell is much more than a combination of molecules and atoms. A cell is a miraculous reality—life itself. A single cell may be a life form, such as a bacterium. A human being, on the other hand, is made of about 75 trillion cells, including about two hundred different kinds of specialized cells with specific functions throughout the body, such as in the brain, the blood, the muscles, the liver and the eyes.

Cells are created and maintained by extremely complex actions and interactions, but nature takes care of that complexity. Your job is rather simple: Make certain that your cells obtain what they need. Choosing health means learning how to supply your cells with what they need while keeping them free of what they don't need. Cells have great powers to take care of themselves and to repair themselves—to stay healthy—unless they are overwhelmed by poor diets, unhealthy habits or environmental hazards. *Your daily choices determine whether your cells stay healthy or get sick.*

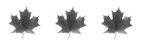

We are ready to begin our journey through the cells of your body. Picture that we have traveled to the largest industrial park you can imagine. Around the park is a security wall designed to keep out intruders, to prevent the loss of essential materials, and to regulate the passage of materials in and out of the park. Inside the park are powerhouses designed to make the energy necessary to keep the park working. These powerhouses, in turn, require fuel, oxygen and other essentials on a round-the-clock basis in order to do their jobs.

Also inside the park are different factories and manufacturing plants that require a continuous supply of energy and raw materials in order to meet their daily quota of finished products. Coordinating all these activities are computer and communication systems that regulate the delivery of raw materials and the removal of wastes, as well as the production, storage and distribution of finished products. All of these systems are based upon a set of design blueprints containing all the information necessary to build a new park.

You have just toured the human cell. Each cell has a wall—the membrane—whose purpose is to keep out toxins, bacteria, viruses and other harmful substances, while still allowing nutrients to reach inside where they are needed. The membrane also prevents healthy and necessary substances from leaking out of the cell, while still allowing waste products to be excreted. Powerhouses in the cell create energy and manufacturing plants make the finished products your body needs, such as neurotransmitters, hormones and antibodies. Your cells also have electrical and communication systems that help to keep everything working in balance. Cells have many important jobs to perform during every second of every day; anything that interferes with these tasks is a threat to health.

Every day hundreds of billions of cells need to be replaced. Building a new cell requires a long list of raw materials, similar to building a new car or a computer. If even one part is missing, the product will be defective, and if many parts are missing, malfunction is guaranteed. As each new cell is created, you are choosing either health or disease, depending on whether the new cells you are building are healthy or not.

You make this choice when you order at a fast-food drive-up

window, when you stay up too late, when you spray cleaning products around your house, when you take your daily vitamin supplement or when you choose to take no supplements. Making a single bad choice here and there is generally not a problem, but when you consistently make bad choices, daily living can wear down your tissues faster than they can be repaired or replaced.

Building and Operating Healthy Cells

To be healthy, each day old cells must be replaced with new ones and each must perform all of its intended functions. Do you know what raw materials you need to build healthy cells? Are you eating the right foods—foods whose calories are packed with the building blocks required to make healthy new cells? Does anyone really believe it is possible to build healthy cells from coffee, donuts, white bread, pasta, potato chips, french fries and ice cream? How many of the raw materials necessary to build and operate healthy cells do these foods contain? The answer is not many, which is one reason that we have so much disease.

A chronic shortage of vitamins, minerals, water, oxygen or other nutrients causes your cells to malfunction. You may be unaware this malfunction is happening, particularly at the early stages, but a chronic shortage of even one nutrient eventually makes you sick. When shortages are chronic, the body stops repairing and self-regulating; cells then deteriorate into a diseased state or die.

Building healthy cells starts in a mother's womb. If an embryo suffers from a shortage of building materials or the presence of toxins, a child born with birth defects may be the result. During pregnancy, certain parts of the fetus are being constructed during specific weeks—such as the brain and nervous system, the circulatory system and the digestive system. If essential raw materials are unavailable at that crucial

time or toxins are present, any of these systems can be
affected, perhaps manifested as heart defects, digestive problems, lower I.Q., attention deficit disorders and so on. We're
not talking about genetic defects here, but defects that result
from building a baby in an unhealthy environment. In extreme
situations, the construction process simply shuts down and the
fetus is naturally aborted—an ever-increasing occurrence in
our society.

A newborn baby's health is the product of the genetic material from the parents *and* the supply of building materials and
presence of toxins (from the mother) during gestation. People
wrongly assume that genetics by itself explains the health or
disease of their child. Congenital defects (those present at
birth) are not necessarily the result of genetics. For example,
the December 2001 issue of *Lancet* reported a study regarding
supplemental vitamins taken during pregnancy. Mothers who
had taken both folic acid and iron supplements during pregnancy gave birth to children who were 60 percent less likely
to develop the most common form of childhood leukemia.
Eating right is especially important for expecting moms. Like
any disease, leukemia doesn't "just happen." The quality of
the cells, tissues and systems a baby is born with has a lifelong
effect.

Whether caused by nutritional deficiency or toxic exposure,
trouble can begin when your cell factories are supposed to be
making something but are not making enough or have shut
down. If cell factories are unable to make sufficient antibodies, we become susceptible to infections. When cell factories
cannot make sufficient neurotransmitters, mental function suffers. (Neurotransmitters are chemicals generated by nerve
cells that send information throughout the nervous system, allowing us to think, learn and remember.) When unable to make
sufficient hormones, communications and self-regulation are
disrupted.

Hormones are chemicals produced by specialized cells that

travel through the blood and lymph systems to bring messages to other parts of the body. Blood sugar level, for instance, is balanced primarily by two hormones, both produced by specialized cells in the pancreas.

Although each cell is a living entity unto itself, bodily systems can only be regulated and controlled when cells are able to communicate effectively with each other. *Impaired cellular communications is one of the most basic common denominators of disease, no matter how the disease happened or what it is called.* Cellular communication and feedback systems regulate everything from body temperature to immunity to movement. When these systems break down gradually, as they often do in disease, we may not notice. We are more familiar with sudden and severe breakdowns in bodily communication, such as spinal injuries that cause paralysis. We fail to recognize how subtle communication breakdowns precipitate chronic and terminal health problems.

Each time you order at a restaurant, each time you reach into your cabinet for cooking oils, each time you plan your day's meals, you are basically deciding whether you will build strong cells or weak ones. It really is that simple. The choice is yours to make. Are you going to maintain your body or let it fall apart?

Toxins Shut Systems Down

A variety of toxic chemicals and metals can damage cells. Like grains of sand, toxins can jam cellular machinery and even cause entire cell factories or powerhouses to shut down.

Many toxins disable enzymes, which are necessary for the chemical reactions that make our lives possible. The number of chemical reactions required to make life possible is astonishing; in a cell, an estimated 6 trillion such reactions take place every second. Enzymes make these reactions possible. About two thousand kinds of enzymes have been identified, and they are manufactured by our cells to accomplish a variety of tasks. Enzymes act as little machines, putting things together or taking them apart at amazingly high speed. Without functioning enzymes, cell factories and assembly lines shut down.

The kind of enzymes a particular cell manufactures distinguishes and determines what kind of cell it is (for example, a nerve cell or a muscle cell). Enzymes serve a variety of purposes and must be constructed with many different nutrients. Enzymes contain essential mineral atoms, such as zinc, magnesium, iron and chromium. If these building materials are not present in sufficient quantity, enzyme function (and therefore cell function) is impaired. Take zinc, for example. The retina contains enzymes constructed with zinc and is a zinc-rich tissue. If you do not have enough zinc in your diet, your retina and other zinc-rich tissues, such as the prostate, will be impaired before obvious effects are noticed elsewhere in the body. Night blindness and malfunctioning prostates are common symptoms of zinc deficiency.

However, even if dietary zinc is adequate, but this nutrient is replaced in the enzyme by a toxic metal—such as mercury, arsenic, cadmium or lead—the presence of this toxin disables the enzyme and causes disease. Toxic heavy metals are a prime example of how toxins can cause cellular malfunction, and our bodies contain hundreds of times more toxic metals than they did in our ancestors a century ago. Mercury is a toxic heavy metal that we are commonly exposed to from dental work—amalgam fillings contain mercury. Municipal water supplies contain toxins such as aluminum, fluoride and arsenic. Even in trace amounts, these toxins can deactivate enzymes and impair vital bodily systems. They can cause our systems to shut down. They must be avoided.

Building and using enzymes properly is an essential part of good health, as enzyme dysfunction is a common denominator of disease. Maintaining proper enzyme balance is one reason to eat fresh organic foods. Organic produce is richer in the vitamins and minerals that enable us to build enzymes and coenzymes, and it is less toxic, too. Enzyme function can also be enhanced with high-quality dietary supplements.

The First Line of Defense

A cell's first line of defense against disease is the cell membrane, the security wall that surrounds the cell and carries out many important functions. Healthy membranes, built from appropriate materials, protect cells from harmful invaders—including viruses. Malfunctioning membranes allow bacteria, viruses, toxins and other harmful substances to damage cells. The presence of poorly constructed cell membranes formed from poor diets is one of the biggest reasons that almost all Americans get sick.

The cell membrane controls everything that goes into and out of a cell. Making certain that only the right things go in and out of the cell is a critical and complex task that only can be accomplished when the cell membrane is constructed correctly. The membranes that surround each of the trillions of cells in your body are made mostly of fats and oils. Membranes constructed out of the wrong fats and oils do not function properly, which is a problem for most Americans. For example, diets with excessive amounts of saturated fats, which are rigid molecules, create rigid cell membranes that lack necessary elasticity. Catastrophic failures, such as ruptured blood vessels and torn muscles and tendons, can occur in tissues made from these rigid cells.

Cell membranes are made primarily of fatty molecules called phospholipids. Special kinds of oils called essential fatty acids (EFAs)—omega-3s and omega-6s—are used to create the phospholipids in cell membranes. These oils are essential because your body is unable to produce them; these oils must be obtained through diet. An overwhelming majority

—some estimate as much as 90 percent—of the U.S. population may be deficient in the correct assortment of essential fatty acids. When the correct raw materials are lacking, the body makes cell membranes out of whatever raw materials are available. These materials include the hydrogenated oils found in margarine, vegetable shortening, baked goods and breakfast cereals; the saturated fats from meat and dairy products; and the trans-fatty acids found in processed salad and cooking oils. Cell membranes built from these inappropriate fats and oils cause the membrane and the entire cell to malfunction.

For example, building a cell membrane from hydrogenated oils impairs the passage of oxygen into the cell, and oxygen-deficient cells become cancerous. None of us would build a house with cardboard walls. Why, then, do we build our cell membranes—our first line of defense against disease—out of junk materials like margarine, vegetable shortening and supermarket oils? Modern diets fail to supply adequate amounts of the correct essential fatty acids. I recommend supplementation with high-quality essential fatty acids and fish oils (see appendix C).

Weak and Rusty

To be healthy, cells must be supplied with adequate amounts of antioxidants. Cell membranes and the factories and powerhouses inside of cells can be damaged from oxidation via free radicals. Picture how oxidative damage (rust) would cause the Golden Gate Bridge to disintegrate were it not painted with a protective coating each year. Currently, our bodies are immersed in a sea of highly reactive chemicals—such as ozone in urban air and chlorine in tap water—that create oxidative damage to our bodies. You likely have heard reports about antioxidants (such as vitamins A, C and E) and how they protect us against free radical damage.

Free radicals damage our cells just like rust corrodes metal. Free radicals have unpaired electrons. Electrons, which travel in pairs, are charged particles orbiting around the nucleus of atoms. An unpaired electron aggressively seeks a mate, trying to "grab" an electron from something else, perhaps a molecule that is performing an important job in one of your cell membranes. Once the electron is grabbed, that molecule can no longer perform its job properly; furthermore, the molecule now becomes a free radical itself, aggressively seeking its own electron mate. The subsequent chain reaction can result in serious cellular damage commonly associated with aging and disease, unless the body's tissues are rich with antioxidants that can stop hazardous chain reactions as soon as they begin.

Free radicals are naturally produced as we metabolize oxygen. Free-radical chain reactions are constantly being produced and stopped inside your body. Cells were designed to cope with these reactions, but not of the magnitude that is present today. For example, chlorine, a highly oxidizing gas put in municipal tap water, can easily damage our skin and lungs. Taking a shower in chlorinated water is like stepping into a chlorine gas chamber—a health hazard of which most people are totally unaware. We can make choices to protect our cells, but first we need to know the source of the damage.

Today, we expose ourselves to free-radical damage from chemicals to which our biological ancestors were never exposed. Our modern environment is filled with substances that cause free radicals to form, such as ozone, chlorine, pesticides, tobacco smoke, petroleum byproducts, synthetic perfume and many others. We need more antioxidant protection than ever, because we are exposed to so many more free radicals. The problem is that the need for antioxidant nutrients is up while the supply in our diet is down.

To avoid the weak and rusty body—to slow the aging process and keep disease at bay—the sensible solution is to stop the free-radical damage. The necessities are simple: a diet rich in antioxidant nutrients along with antioxidant supplements, and clean food, water and air. None of these ideas are new, but what people don't understand is why they are important. If you allow free radicals to damage your cells—to allow them to become weak and rusty—your body ages faster and becomes vulnerable to disease.

Salt Is Often at Fault

To be healthy, the nutrients in cells must be in proper balance. Upsetting the natural balance of chemicals inside a cell causes the cell to malfunction, which is what is happening to the balance of sodium and potassium in our cells. Over the past one hundred years, our diets have changed dramatically, increasing the amount of sodium and decreasing the amount of potassium in our diet, thus reversing the natural balance. Modern food manufacturers add lots of salt (sodium chloride) to their products, while modern diets do not include enough potassium-rich foods such as fresh fruits, vegetables, whole grains and legumes. When our genes were evolving, human diets contained little sodium and a lot of potassium. For example, eating an apple provides only 1 mg of sodium, but 310 mg of potassium. Eating a piece of modern apple pie provides 110 mg of sodium and only 80 mg of potassium, a drastic change.

Salt-rich diets force excess sodium into cells, disturbing the normal and healthy sodium/potassium balance. Among other problems, excess sodium interferes with cellular energy production, causing fatigue. Sodium attaches itself strongly to water molecules, so when more sodium goes into the cells, so does more water. Water retention elevates blood pressure and causes weight gain. Dietary salt contributes to an increased incidence of cancer and metastasis, cardiac disease, stroke, kidney disease, bronchial problems and kidney stones. By avoiding processed and packaged foods, most of our excess dietary sodium can be eliminated.

An Important Litmus Test

Healthy cells must have the correct pH. In addition to the dangerous imbalance of sodium and potassium, our modern lifestyles and diets have detrimental effects on another critical balance: the pH of our cells. Commercials commonly tout "pH balanced" shampoos for our hair, and most of us remember the litmus paper tests from our chemistry sets or grade-school experiments—those tiny sheets of paper that turn pink or blue based on pH. Cells must maintain proper pH balance, and our food choices affect that balance.

The pH is a measurement of acidity or alkalinity. On the pH scale, 7 is neutral; 0 to 7 is acidic, and 7 to 14 is alkaline. The normal pH inside of a cell is about 7.4, which is slightly alkaline. Maintaining normal pH in the fluid inside the cell as well as in other body fluids is critical for keeping body systems functioning normally. Most of the chemical reactions in the body, including the production of energy, occur most efficiently in an alkaline environment. The enzymes involved in these reactions are pH sensitive and only function within a narrow pH range; pH level affects other vital operations, such as the transport of substances through cell membranes. You can monitor your acid/alkaline levels by using pH paper (see appendix C).

Modern diets often cause cellular pH to drop below 7.0, into the acidic range. (Cells also can become too alkaline, but excessive acidity is most common.) A cell that becomes too acidic is said to have intracellular acidosis. Acidosis, an extremely serious condition, is one of the common factors present in many manifestations of disease. The more acidic a cell becomes, the more impaired its function. At very high acidic levels, the cell will die. Herman Aihara, author of *Acid and Alkaline,* says that "one of the important causes of cancer—and other degenerative diseases—is the cumulative effect of the acidic condition of body fluid."

How do cells become too acidic? Different foods have different effects on our pH. Ideally, we should consume only foods that maintain proper cellular pH. Instead, we consume a diet high in foods that have an acidic effect, such as sugar, soft drinks, white flour (pasta and bread), excessive protein and salt. Consumption of these foods, which deplete the body of alkaline materials, has skyrocketed over the past few generations.

Because acidosis is such a threat, the body tries to prevent it by using its own alkaline minerals (such as calcium and magnesium) leached from the bones and teeth, leading to dental problems and osteoporosis. By contrast, fresh and unprocessed foods, rich in alkaline minerals, help keep pH within normal limits. For this reason, among others, most of our calories should come from fresh, unprocessed vegetables, fruits, beans and whole grains.

Concerned about your pH? Measure the pH of your first morning urine before eating. This test offers an indicator of your cellular pH and can be used to monitor changes as you work to normalize your pH. First morning urine should be in the range of 6.5 to 7.5. If readings fall below 6.5, you are too acidic. Occasional readings above 7.5 are normal, but consistent readings above 7.5 are an indication of tissue breakdown, and a pH over 8.0 is a serious matter. Fatigue is often reflected in an acidic pH.

Why Am I So Tired?

Fatigue is one of the most common complaints made to physicians today. During the onset of my own illness, the first thing I noticed was fatigue. I simply did not have the energy I had been accustomed to having. So many people—epidemic proportions, actually—are tired and lack energy, but they do not know what to do about it. Indeed, when I told my doctor about my fatigue, he told me it was the result of aging. In truth, the fatigue had nothing to do with growing older and everything to do with becoming sicker.

All cells require energy to function. Your cellular power-houses use enzymes to turn carbohydrates, fatty acids and amino acids into energy the body is able to use. Fatigue occurs because the body's energy production systems have been impaired. The powerhouses (called *mitochondria*) may not be receiving sufficient fuel or oxygen, may have been damaged by free radicals, may have the wrong pH, or may have their enzymes disabled by toxic chemicals. The high-energy compounds made by the powerhouses, such as ATP (adenosine triphosphate), are made in large quantities when we sleep, which is one reason that an under-rested person functions poorly and lacks energy.

Don't Blame Your Parents

Genes are the blueprints for the structure and function of every cell in our bodies. Although we inherit genes from our parents, how we maintain and care for our genes determines how well our cells work. Over a lifetime, to some degree, genes deteriorate and mutate naturally, but what we must focus on are man-made free radicals that accelerate or distort this natural process. Minimizing the damage is crucial; important steps are to avoid: radiation from medical X rays and other sources, environmental chemicals, prescription and recreational drugs, alcohol, tobacco smoke and even char-broiled meat. Minimizing the damage also means protecting genes with good nutrition—particularly foods containing ample antioxidant nutrients such as vitamins A, C, E and the mineral selenium.

Many people assume that "bad genes" or a family history of disease predestines them to be sick. In truth, while genetic predispositions do put a person at risk for disease, what a person chooses to do to protect the health of their cells and genes plays a more important role in whether or not disease develops. Choices, rather than genetic inheritance, are the key. We must focus on how we play the game, not the cards we were dealt; what we eat, what we do and what we are exposed to determines how healthy we will be.

Learning a New Way

Unfortunately, a common medical response to a diseased organ is to remove it surgically. Before taking such a drastic action, why not give the cells that make up that organ what they need, keep them free of what they do not need and restore the organ to health?

Modern lifestyles—diets and toxins—create the formulas for cellular malfunction and disease, yet traditional medical practices ignore them. How often have you, a friend or a relative consulted a physician and been given a diagnosis or treatment but were not asked even one question about how you care for or neglect your body? Not asked even one question about what you eat, what harmful substances invade your environment or how you live your life in general? More commonly you are asked about symptoms alone. Traditional medicine does not make us healthy and, worse yet, can make us sick and promote our death. Drugs, surgeries and other medical procedures that disregard the causes of disease—not fixing the problems inside the cells and instead addressing symptoms—can never cure the disease. Disease is not about "diseases," it is about cells; diagnoses and treatments should always reflect this approach.

The battle between sickness and health takes place within every cell in your body. Choosing healthy cells means following each of the six pathways in a positive direction; let us move on to the first of the six: the nutrition pathway.

5

THE NUTRITION PATHWAY

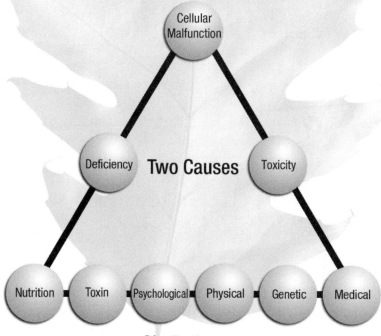

One Disease

Cellular Malfunction

Deficiency   Two Causes   Toxicity

Nutrition   Toxin   Psychological   Physical   Genetic   Medical

Six Pathways

"The well-nourished American is a myth. Despite the high level of education and the abundance of available food, many people make poor food choices and are badly nourished. . . . [T]he average human diet, nutritionally unfit for rats, must be equally unsatisfactory or even more so in meeting human needs."

Carl Pfeiffer, M.D., Ph.D.
Mental and Elemental Nutrients

Meet Elizabeth. For eight years Elizabeth has waged a losing battle against chronic fatigue. She suffers from painful arthritis (with measurable bone loss in one shoulder), and she takes powerful pain medications daily. Overwhelming exhaustion, coupled with the pain, prevent her from working or participating in meaningful activity. She has seen numerous medical doctors and alternative practitioners, but she is not improving.

After hearing me speak at a chronic fatigue support group, Elizabeth reached out for my help. Within a few months Elizabeth's pain was gone and her energy was soaring. A year later, she returned to work, at a six-figure income. "Raymond gave me back my life," she tells friends. In reality, I simply taught her how to give her cells the nutrients they were desperately missing. Even more simply, I taught Elizabeth how to shop for food, prepare meals and find high-quality vitamin supplements. Simple, essential and life-saving.

To become healthier, Elizabeth began to consume more nutritious foods, eat more raw foods and fewer cooked ones. She was careful about which foods to combine together. She cut back on sugar, white flour, hydrogenated oils and milk products, as well as coffee. These choices literally made Elizabeth a changed woman; her whole life and health were turned around by improving the chemistry inside her cells. Her fatigue and arthritis pain gradually disappeared, and she actually repaired much of the damaged bone tissue in her arthritic shoulder.

In various forms, Elizabeth's story of declining health is played out millions of times each day in this country. Few Americans go to bed hungry, but almost all Americans go to bed malnourished, some severely so. This concept may be difficult to accept because we typically envision malnourished third-world people with distended bellies and listless eyes. In truth, "well-fed" Americans, including those—or perhaps especially those—who are overweight, are "starving" for the kinds of food needed to become and stay healthy.

Most of us eat the wrong foods. I call them "make-believe" foods that do not meet the needs of our cells. In fact, 90 percent of the typical American food budget is spent on make-believe foods. Most of us spend lots of money and lots of time shopping for and preparing meals that are, in small and large ways, killing our cells, creating disease and shortening our lives.

We shop in supermarkets full of empty-calorie foods. We buy foods that have been so mishandled that they no longer offer the nutrition we think we are buying. We prepare and cook our foods in ways that destroy their nutritional value. Nearly all of us—from junk-food junkies to "health-conscious" consumers—are being misled into believing that low-fat products and typical supermarket meat and produce can build a healthy diet. Consider:

- Too much of our diet is created from an officially approved "Big Four" list of foods that fail to nurture our bodies and also create toxins that sicken us. The Big Four? Sugar, white flour, processed oils and milk products. Even foods touted as "healthy," such as multigrain breads, usually contain impoverished flour.

- We eat the cells of unhealthy plants and animals, which cannot create healthy cells in our body. Pigs and other livestock are fed toxic diets. Chemicals used during growing, harvesting, processing, transporting and storing diminish nutrients in produce. In no way can such food support our cell chemistry.

- Too little of our food—virtually none for many people—is eaten raw. Cooking damages foods' nutritional values. Some cooking methods, particularly those that use high heat or that char foods, create powerful mutagens and carcinogens.

- Handling and preparation methods—from extended storing of foods in a refrigerator or freezer to chopping and mashing—rob foods of many nutrients such as vitamins and minerals that we believe we are consuming. The average person preparing a meal damages and destroys the power of the food, even food the individual considers to be "fresh."

- Commercial practices used to supply food from farms to supermarkets are overwhelmingly destructive. Produce is often harvested before it is ripe, stored for long periods of time and subjected to harmful methods to ripen or color it artificially for presentation in the "fresh" produce section of the supermarket. Some of this produce has lost nearly all of certain vitamins and minerals by the time it rolls down the supermarket checkout lines, let alone by the time we eat it.

- The way we eat our foods—even how we chew—often prevents us from realizing the best nutrition, even from good diets. We also eat the wrong combinations of foods, which interfere with effective digestion.
- Most of the vitamin and mineral supplements sold today are of poor quality and not worth what you pay for them. They do not provide us with the nutrients we think we are buying.

Starvation on a Full Stomach

According to the *State of the World 2000* report from the Worldwatch Institute, the world is in the midst of a nutrition crisis. In the developed countries, 1.2 billion people, including most Americans, are now "starving" and undernourished because they are overfed with too much of the wrong foods. The average American diet does not support the biological needs of human cells. We try to achieve the impossible: We try to maintain health while eating a diet that cannot provide health. Although our stomachs may be full (and our bellies are fat), malnutrition is our leading cause of disease.

Ultimately, any level of malnutrition creates susceptibility to disease. However, when we suffer health problems as a result of poor nutrition, almost always we blame our illnesses on aging or on faulty genes rather than on its true cause.

We are, indeed, what we eat. That cliché should guide all choices we make about the foods we consume. The average person, however, is poorly informed and confused about what to eat, how to eat and what to avoid. Misinformation tossed about by food manufacturers and even by physicians overwhelms the consumer. Few people truly understand how food helps or fails to keep them healthy.

Food manufacturers nearly always favor qualities such as shelf life, taste, appearance and marketability over nutrition and health. Physicians, who typically lack nutrition education themselves, usually tell us that a standard diet gives us all the nutrition we need. With such misinformation, we tend to make irrational and harmful decisions. A diet that focuses on anything other than meeting the nutritional needs of cells allows your body to get sick.

The four worst food choices, comprising the bulk of the average American diet and disastrous to the health of our population are:

1. *sugar*
2. *white flour*
3. *processed oils*
4. *milk products*

Consuming these foods, especially as a large part of the diet and over time, is virtually guaranteed to cause disease. They provide little nutrition and are toxic as well. If every American were to stop eating these "foods," our epidemic of chronic diseases would decline dramatically. Problematic in their own right, the real harm caused by these four food failures comes from the fact that we eat them repeatedly, day by day, meal by meal.

As highly as we might think of ourselves, on a physical level we are nothing more than an organized mass of about 75 trillion cells, all constantly demanding nutrients. If we consistently choose the Big Four—sugar, white flour, processed oils, milk products or foods containing these as ingredients—we cannot hope to meet the needs of our hungry cells. Every single time you choose an organic, fresh, unprocessed food instead of one of the Big Four, you are doing your cells (and yourself) a great service. Let us have a closer look at the Big Four.

Sugar Wreaks Havoc

If you make only one change in your diet, let it be to eliminate or at least reduce your intake of sugar.

People in our society eat an enormous amount of sugar—probably far more than you realize. As is often the case, our perspective is the real problem; we are so familiar with sugar that we do not think of it as a serious health threat. Furthermore, because in one form or another sugar is contained in an enormous number of processed foods, it is almost impossible to avoid.

Sugar even in small amounts is detrimental. Just two teaspoons of sugar (far less than a typical soft drink or bowl of breakfast cereal) has a significant hormonal and nutritional impact for several hours, throwing the body out of balance and into a state of biochemical chaos. If you eat sugar morning, noon and night (as many people do), your body remains in chaos all day, every day. In this state of chaos your body constantly tries to restore its balance but never quite succeeds. Sugar is so damaging to body chemistry that, in his 2000 book, *Fit for Life: A New Beginning,* Harvey Diamond calls refined sugar "a deadly, virulent poison."

During many thousands of years of human evolution, our ancestors survived fine without any sugar other than sugars naturally occurring in wild fruits and berries. Refined sugar is a comparatively recent invention, and only very recently has it become a dietary staple. In 1750, when it was first introduced to North America, sugar was a rare and expensive commodity, and even in 1900 the average person ate only 10 pounds of sugar per year. By 1985, sugar consumption had risen to 124 pounds per year, and by the year 2000 the average American ate a whopping 160 pounds of sugar per year! Most of us cannot comprehend eating this much sugar because we fail to realize that it is in almost every type of processed food. The average American now consumes about one quarter of his or her calories from sugar, and many children receive almost half of their calories from sugar.

All the calories from sugar are empty calories, containing virtually none of the nutrients that your cells need so desperately. Furthermore, sugar is an antinutrient; *eating sugar drains nutrients from your body.* Certain nutrients (which are present in raw sugarcane but not in refined sugar) are needed for you to metabolize the sugar. Your body must obtain these nutrients from somewhere, and because they are not in the sugar they are robbed from your own tissues—thereby depleting your health.

Sugar consumption contributes not only to the more obvious health problems such as diabetes and tooth decay, but also to heart disease, osteoporosis and immune dysfunction. If you want to avoid colds or if someone in your family is "coming down with a cold," eliminate sugar.

Our society constantly worries about the relationship between high-cholesterol animal products and heart disease, yet sugar is a more serious cause. A study by A. M. Cohen, M.D., published in a 1961 issue of the medical journal *Lancet,* reports that Jews from Yemen were noted to have very little heart disease, even though the diet in Yemen is typically high in animal fat. When these Jews moved to Israel, where a lot of sugar is common in the diet, rates of heart disease increased dramatically.

Being an antinutrient, sugar also causes calcium to be lost in the urine, forcing the body to remove calcium from the bones in order to keep the blood calcium levels within normal limits. By taking the calcium out of your bones, eating sugar contributes to osteoporosis. People concerned about or already suffering from osteoporosis should eliminate sugar from their diet.

Eating sugar causes deficiencies of a number of minerals, including calcium, chromium, magnesium and zinc. When you do not have enough minerals, your body has difficulty producing sufficient digestive enzymes needed for good digestion. Undigested food particles can enter into your bloodstream, creating serious problems such as allergies and immune-deficiency diseases. This is why foods consumed with sugar (such as wheat, corn, milk and eggs) become the most common allergens. If you enjoy your foods and do not want to become allergic to them, learn to avoid combining them with sugar.

In this modern age of AIDS, autoimmune and other immune system diseases, sugar creates special problems. Sugar damages the cells of our immune system, creating susceptibility to colds, flu and other immune-related diseases. Sugar also plays a crucial role in the development of diabetes. The mechanisms for controlling blood sugar become faulty when high levels of sugar are present in the diet. Sugar also causes a calcium/phosphorous imbalance, which makes the body less capable of breaking proteins down into the amino acids that are required to make essential body chemicals. Even traditional doctors acknowledge that sugar causes tooth decay. Historically, natives who had little exposure to the civilized world and refined sugar had almost no tooth decay.

Sugar is bad enough by itself, but also it is a dangerous partner. You should especially avoid combining sugar with protein (such as a sweet dessert after a steak dinner, or orange juice with eggs in the morning). In combination, they react and form damaging compounds called AGEs (advanced glycation end products). AGEs may even form within your foods before you eat them, if sugar and protein are cooked together (such as baked goods containing eggs and sugar, or a ham baked with brown sugar on top). These AGEs are known to promote heart disease, high blood pressure, cataracts and arthritis.

Eating refined sugar is destructive to human health because it causes vitamins, minerals and hormones to become imbalanced, which throws the body into biochemical chaos for several hours. The body, desperately scrambling to right itself, depletes itself of vital nutrients. The most important and universal dietary recommendation I can make to everyone is to cut as much sugar (and foods made with sugar) from their diet as possible. Those children who are consuming up to half their calories as sugar become sitting ducks for infections and future problems such as diabetes, osteoporosis, cancer, arthritis and heart disease. Eating sugar is death by installment.

White Flour: Quick, Inexpensive and Destructive

Almost all bread, pasta and baked goods are made of white flour—an easy-to-use, easy-to-store, highly processed derivative of what was once a wheat grain. Wheat is a good and nutritious food, but by the time wheat gets ground up and processed into white flour, it bears little resemblance (physically or nutritionally) to wheat. White flour contains little nutrition, is toxic and is an antinutrient (like sugar). Yet the average American consumes more than two hundred pounds of white flour every year.

Almost all of the nutrients once contained in wheat are lost in the process of creating white flour (including 60 percent of the calcium, 77 percent of the magnesium, 78 percent of the zinc, 89 percent of the cobalt, 98 percent of the vitamin E, 80 percent of vitamins B_1 and B_3, and 75 percent of the folic acid). Also lost are the essential fatty acids and fiber. Worse still, many nutrients are needed in order for your body to metabolize the flour for energy. Because the flour does not contain those nutrients, your body is robbed of the nutrients, similar to what happens when you eat sugar.

In 1941, severe nutritional problems prompted our government to pass legislation requiring that certain nutrients be added back to the flour. "Enriched flour" was born. White flour has lost more than twenty-five known nutrients, a handful are added back, yet we still call flour "enriched" (instead of, perhaps, "impoverished").

We did not have nutritional deficiency in mind when we

started making white flour. We made it because it does not spoil; it keeps practically forever, which makes white flour an ideal food to feed people in big cities. However, the malnutrition problem with flour is serious—our bellies are filled in the form of "hearty" pastas and breads, but all those empty calories do not even come close to fulfilling our needs for nutrients, thus contributing to deficiency.

Worse, flour also contributes to the other cause of disease, toxicity. White flour contains almost no fiber, which is essential for proper bowel movements and toxin removal. Eating too much flour (and not enough fiber) is associated with constipation, hemorrhoids, colitis and rectal cancer.

Avoiding white flour is not easy because it is in virtually all breads, pastas, cakes, cookies, crackers, breakfast cereals, pizzas and pastries. But when you realize that flour causes disease, cutting down on the refined flour products you consume is worth the effort. A plate of pasta with vegetables can no longer be considered a good meal. The vegetables are good, but the pasta is not; choose whole grains or beans instead.

The real health threat from white flour comes not from any single meal, but because we eat so much of it—one or more meals a day, every day. We also need to keep in mind that many other grains frequently are refined (such as those in "multigrain" breads and cereals) and are reduced to little more than empty calories. Any grain that is finely ground and "stripped" of fiber and other nutrients is a poor nutritional choice because essential nutrients have been lost, which most people do not realize. I cannot tell you how many times I have talked to people who proudly describe their "healthy, whole-grain diets"—diets made of whole-wheat bread, rolled oats, granola, multigrain cereals. All of these are processed, make-believe foods. *Eating processed foods of any kind is fundamentally different from and nutritionally inferior to eating whole, unprocessed foods.*

On the subject of food processing, one type of grain processing is of special concern: puffed grains. The high heat and

pressure used in the puffing process alters the molecular structure of proteins in the grains, making them toxic enough to kill
laboratory animals. Absolutely avoid puffed wheat, puffed
millet and puffed rice (including rice cakes), and any other
puffed grains. This warning does not include popcorn, which
is not subjected to such high temperatures and pressures. In
his book, *Fighting the Food Giants,* Paul Stitt reported an
experiment in which rats were fed either whole wheat or
puffed wheat. The rats eating the whole wheat lived over a
year while the rats eating puffed wheat died within two weeks.

To avoid health problems created by processed grains,
choose whole grains such as millet, oats, quinoa, spelt, barley,
amaranth, teff, kamut and brown rice. Many people do not
realize that white rice is also a processed grain and, therefore,
a poor food choice. Buckwheat, not strictly a grain, can be
cooked like whole grains. Organic whole grains are readily
available at health food stores. Cook grains in a pot of water
as you would cook rice. A rice-cooker will also work. In the
real world, often we are forced to make less than ideal choices.
At the very least, choose minimally processed whole grains
(such as whole-wheat flour or oatmeal) instead of highly
refined and stripped grains, such as white flour, white rice and
pasta made from white flour.

Misleading Choices

When I told Elizabeth, the woman I introduced you to at the
start of this chapter, that if she wanted to get well and stay well
she would have to eliminate sugar from her diet, she replied,
"I don't eat any sugar," going on to explain that she rarely
added sugar to anything. What she meant was, she rarely took
white sugar out of the sugar bowl and added it to her foods and
beverages. She was not considering the massive amounts of
sugar already present in her diet from foods as mundane as
ketchup, breakfast cereal, dinner rolls, soup, salad dressing,
bottled fruit juices and soft drinks, not to mention chocolates,

ice cream, cookies, pies, cakes, snack foods and pancake syrup. Elizabeth was quite surprised when I added up all the sugar she was consuming.

Elizabeth and I also talked about white flour. She did not realize that most of the starches she was eating (including pastas, breads and breakfast cereals) were made from white flour and other processed grains. Thinking about what she should perhaps be eating instead, she made another mistake: Elizabeth proudly showed me a package of the "healthy" multigrain bread she had purchased. I shook my head as I read the ingredient list and explained to her that such bread is not healthy. First, bread is a highly processed food, and this bread's number-one ingredient was unbleached flour, a highly processed flour that is only marginally better than white flour (it has not undergone the final bleaching process). This supposedly "healthy" bread also contained a health-damaging sugar (corn syrup), hydrogenated oils and toxic preservatives.

Elizabeth had been misled into believing this bread was a healthy food—perhaps because of the false advertising on the package, claiming it to be "healthy," and the fact that she had purchased it in a health food store. Many people have a difficult time learning how to discern good foods from bad ones. The simplest explanation is to think of the concepts of *real foods* and *make-believe foods*. The more a food is changed from the way nature would normally provide it, the more make-believe it becomes.

Some Truths about Processed Fats and Oils

A widespread misperception in America today is that to be healthy we must eat a low-cholesterol, low-fat or nonfat diet. Rather, you need fats and oils, but they must be the right kinds of fats and oils, not the processed fats and oils so prevalent in our diets today. Despite our society's obsession with and fears about fats and oils, these nutrients are an incredibly important part of a healthy diet.

Each of the trillions of cells in your body is surrounded by a permeable cell membrane. Fats and oils are the primary building materials used to create those cell membranes. Cell membranes are critically important because all the nutrients your cells need and all the toxic waste products they must eliminate need to pass through it. If you eat the right kinds of fats and oils, your cell membranes properly regulate the passage of materials; eating the wrong kinds causes your cell membranes to work against you. When your cell membranes are not working correctly, your cells will malfunction, which can manifest into just about any disease you can imagine.

Essential fatty acids is the term used to describe the "right kind" of fats and oils. They are essential because the body needs them but cannot make them, so we must obtain them from food. These essential fatty acid molecules have a specific shape that is critical to the way they work in forming cell membranes—like bricks that fit perfectly together to build cell walls. (Chemists use the term cis-fatty acids to describe the natural, healthy shape of essential fatty acid molecules.)

When oils are heated above 392°F (as most supermarket oils are), the cis-fatty acid molecules change shape, turning into a different and toxic category of fats called trans-fats. The shape of trans-fats does not work properly for building cell membranes. These improperly shaped "bricks" build a cell wall with holes it. Cell membranes constructed from trans-fats become leaky (allowing substances inside cells to leak out, and vice versa) and brittle (like the shell of an egg, rather than the elasticity of a balloon). If cells throughout your body are leaky and brittle, you have a serious problem.

Because of the way oils are processed, trans-fats (and other toxins) are found in virtually all oils sold in supermarkets and health food stores, including canola, corn, safflower, sunflower, cottonseed and soybean oils, along with food products containing hydrogenated oils, like margarine and vegetable shortenings. Consider the vast numbers of products made with these toxic oils, such as salad dressings, breakfast cereals, crackers, chocolates, candy, potato chips and fried foods such as french fries. The solution? Eat essential (good) fats and avoid hydrogenated and other (bad) trans-fats.

More chemistry that is vital to your health: The two most important essential fatty acids are linoleic acid (omega-6 fatty acids) and linolenic acid (omega-3 fatty acids). For good health, these fatty acids must be consumed in sufficient amounts and in the correct balance with each other. It has been estimated, however, that 60 percent of our population gets too much omega-6s and that up to 95 percent gets too little omega-3s; this imbalance causes disease. Avoid processed, supermarket oils and food products containing them, which perpetuate this imbalance, and supplement with oils combining a healthy balance.

Pioneers in medical research are curing a number of chronic problems (such as depression, heart disease and cancer) by giving their patients the right kinds of fats and oils. But most people have no idea that the bad fats and oils damage cell membranes and therefore cause disease, which explains why society at large is not demanding alternatives.

As with many of our modern foods, we created technologies that are solely designed to produce the highest amount of oils using the smallest amount of raw materials (seeds, beans and grains) in the shortest period of time with maximum shelf life. Time and money are the driving forces, not health and nutrition. Today, oils are extracted using huge, powerful presses that generate a lot of heat, which, in the presence of oxygen, oxidizes oils, making them rancid and toxic. Yet these now-toxic oils can still be labeled as "cold-pressed" because no heat was added during the pressing process; the heat is an unintentional result of the high-pressure extraction process. *This is why cold-pressed is a meaningless term and is not useful for you in determining what to eat and what to avoid.* Harsh solvents are used to extract oils, which remain in the oil as a residue. These solvents also destroy nutrients in the oils. In addition, processed oils are typically bleached and deodorized—destroying more nutrients and creating toxins.

To put healthful oils in your diet, eat high-quality olive oil and flaxseed oil. Also, beneficial fatty acids can be found in organic, fresh, unprocessed food in its natural state, such as raw seeds, raw nuts and avocados. High-quality eggs, meat and fish are also good sources of fatty acids. Keep in mind, though, that essential fatty acids are readily damaged by heat. Use the minimum heat necessary to cook these foods. Supplement your diet with a high-quality essential fatty acid supplement. *To avoid chronic disease and slow down the aging process, dietary supplementation of essential fatty acids (from flaxseed oil, for example) is necessary; deriving enough of the right fats and oils from the foods that are available today is difficult.*

Check your kitchen and refrigerator shelves. Discard your processed oils, particularly hydrogenated and partially hydrogenated oils (margarine, vegetable shortening, etc.), and products made with those oils, including many baked goods, crackers, chips, peanut butter and nondairy creamer. Instead, use primarily high-quality olive oil, organic butter or ghee, and essential fatty acid supplements (see appendix C for suggestions).

Myths About Milk

The final failure food on my Big Four list is one that is usually touted as necessary to good health for adults and children: milk products. Milk's reputation as a highly nutritious food is undeserved; in reality, modern milk is a highly toxic and allergenic make-believe food. The United States may produce a lot of milk, and the dairy boards may try to convince us to drink lots of milk, but milk does not do a body good.

According to pediatrician Russell Bunai, M.D., in a 1994 issue of *Natural Health,* the one single change to the U.S. diet that could provide the greatest health benefits is the elimination of milk products. In the 1992 edition of his book *Don't Drink Your Milk,* Dr. Frank Oski, former director of the Department of Pediatrics at Johns Hopkins University School of Medicine, said, "We should all stop drinking milk. . . . It was designed for calves, not for humans." This claim is not what your mother told you (because she herself was misled), and it is not what the dairy industry would have you believe, but it is true. The idea that milk is a necessary and healthy part of the human diet is a myth. As I lecture across the country, recommending (among other things) that people not drink milk, I am always amazed at how many times people will call me months later to say that they took my advice, stopped consuming dairy products, and their health problems disappeared.

Most of the world's population (about 70 percent) does not drink milk or consume other dairy products (including cheese, yogurt, ice cream and sour cream), for good reasons. Mother's milk is a perfect food—for infants, not for adults. In nature, no animal drinks milk after weaning, nor does any species drink the milk of another species. Granted, we humans have managed to domesticate our livestock, but this accomplishment does not change the fact that each species (and their milk) is unique. Feeding elephant milk to cats, mouse milk to giraffes or cow milk to humans is not a good idea.

Cow milk, especially in the forms found in your supermarket, is not a good food. Cow milk contains proteins and fats that are difficult for humans to digest, and cow milk does not supply nearly the amount of calcium that its reputation suggests. Also, statistics from the World Health Organization show that the countries consuming the most milk products also have the highest rates of osteoporosis, breast cancer, allergies and diabetes.

Actually milk can deplete nutrients from our bodies—acting as an antinutrient, just like sugar and white flour. Metabolizing some of the fats in milk (particularly when the milk is pasteurized, and virtually all of it is) uses up essential fatty acids, one of our most serious nutritional deficiencies. For all these reasons, foods containing pasteurized milkfats are at the top of the list of "foods to be avoided." Additionally, if pasteurized milkfats are not properly metabolized (because of an essential fatty acid deficiency, which most Americans have), then the fat may be deposited in arteries, contributing to cardiovascular diseases.

A prime factor contributing to the health problems caused by milk is pasteurization (heating), which both destroys nutrients and creates toxins, thereby contributing to each of the two causes of disease. Animals fed pasteurized milk exhibit poor skeletal development, weak bones, osteoporosis and tooth decay. Calves fed raw milk remain healthy, but calves fed pasteurized milk typically die within eight weeks! If a calf cannot benefit from pasteurized milk, how can a human?

The Rest of the Story

Upon hearing that they should not drink milk, people invariably ask, "How will I be able to get enough calcium if I don't drink milk?" My response is, "Where does a cow, a horse, or an elephant get its calcium?" They get it from plants, which are rich in all kinds of minerals—including calcium. Dark green vegetables such as broccoli, chard and kale are rich sources of absorbable calcium.

Cow milk is also rich in calcium, containing about 1,200 mg of calcium per quart while human milk contains about 300 mg. However, an infant absorbs far more calcium from a quart of human milk than from a quart of cow milk, even though human milk contains less calcium. Cow milk contains a lot of phosphorous, which prevents calcium absorption. Also, cow milk is low in magnesium, which humans need in order to utilize calcium. In short, your body is not able to use the large amount of calcium present in cow milk. You do not use the calcium, so instead it can build up and form kidney stones, bone spurs, gout and atherosclerotic plaque.

Milk robs calcium from bones. The protein in cow milk metabolizes to strong acids, which can be harmful, so instead the body uses the calcium to neutralize those acids—thereby robbing your bones and other tissues in the process. The United States, with only 4 percent of the world's population, consumes more dairy foods than the other 96 percent combined. If milk is really good for our bones, then we should have the strongest bones in the world. Instead, we have one of the highest osteoporosis rates in the world. We are not alone; all other countries with high dairy consumption also have high levels of osteoporosis.

A large percentage of the population is allergic to milk and dairy products, regardless of whether they realize it. Allergic reactions tax the immune system and lower resistance to infections and diseases. Milk allergies are the primary cause of ear infections in children. Given that constant allergic responses shorten your life (and constant use of allergy medications will, too), the answer is to avoid things you are allergic to in the first place. For most people, this means avoiding milk products. According to Dr. Oski, "At least 50 percent of all children are allergic to dairy."

Milk is harmful to young children for another reason: It may trigger childhood diabetes in genetically susceptible children. More recently, milk has been linked to multiple sclerosis. Milk also causes localized inflammations in an infant's intestines and can result in low-level bleeding and iron-deficiency anemia. Because of the problems with allergies, anemia and diabetes, in 1992 the American Academy of Pediatrics recommended that cow milk not be given to babies during their first year of life because it damages health. Yet many mothers are not heeding this advice and still feed their children milk, thinking it is healthy. In September 1992, Benjamin Spock, M.D., (the famous "baby doctor") lent his voice to the growing chorus warning against the dangers of cow's milk, urging parents to use breast milk exclusively. Breast milk, yes; cow's milk, no. Infants should be breast-fed for at least one, and preferably for two to three years. After that, no milk should be consumed.

Our hunter-gatherer ancestors nursed their young for an average of three years, as compared to modern Americans, who nurse for an average of only three months. Introduction of infant feeding formulas has had a negative effect on children's health. Breast-fed infants are less likely to develop inflammatory bowel disease when they become adults than bottle-fed infants. Adults who were breast-fed as infants develop fewer allergies throughout life (even among people whose parents had a history of allergies).

Coffee: A Boost with a Big Price

In addition to the Big Four failures, one more dietary habit is worth mentioning because of its huge negative impact on health: drinking coffee. Coffee is popular because our society chronically suffers low energy and fatigue. The stimulating effects of coffee are used "to get through the day," and they create dependency. The caffeine does not create or sustain long-term energy; it just hypes the system by overstimulating the adrenal glands, which ultimately carries a long-term price. Caffeine increases the amount of sugar in the blood and provides an energy lift, but it also throws body chemistry out of balance.

By doing so, coffee damages health in many ways. Coffee is acidic and contributes to overacidity in the American diet, changing the pH of our cells (and requiring calcium to be robbed from tissues to neutralize the acidity). A number of studies have linked caffeine to urinary calcium loss, which contributes to osteoporosis, hip fractures and death.

One of those studies, printed in a January 1994 issue of the *Journal of the American Medical Association,* found that women who drank two cups of coffee per day increased their risk of hip fracture by 69 percent. Coffee has also been linked to cancer. Coffee that is roasted forms a compound called 3,4-benzopyrene, a powerful carcinogen; an average cup of coffee contains 500 micrograms of known carcinogens. In 1981, professor Brian MacMahon of the Harvard School of Public Health concluded that coffee drinking was the cause of 50 percent of all pancreatic cancer, and that drinking three cups a day increased the risk of pancreatic cancer threefold.

Why we drink so much coffee is easy to understand. We eat the Big Four all the time, which causes our cells to function poorly and produce low energy levels. Then, we have deadlines to meet and schedules to keep, and coffee seems the only means to make it happen. Eat real food and eliminate "make-believe" food, and you may find that your "need" for coffee declines.

Nutrition Is Not in the Eyes of the Beholder

Make-believe food lacks sufficient nutrients because it is highly processed, heavily cooked or commercially farmed. Yet because we grew up eating these foods, we are completely accustomed to them.

Within my lifetime, the practice of eating more make-believe foods instead of organic, fresh, unprocessed foods has increased enormously. For most of my life I lived in areas never more than twenty miles from an apple farm where, during harvest season, I could purchase fresh apples. Today, finding fresh apples is difficult, because most that are for sale have been in long-term storage since harvesting.

Produce such as apples, cucumbers, bell peppers and tomatoes are waxed to prevent loss of moisture during long-term storage; this wax is not good for you and often seals in toxic pesticide and fungicide residues as well.

Modern eggs are another example of make-believe food. A real egg contains a fatty acid called DHA (docosahexanoic acid), a nutrient that is a critical building component for cells in brain and eye tissue. A real egg supplies an average of 200 to 400 milligrams of DHA. Make-believe supermarket eggs contain an average of only 18 milligrams. Without adequate DHA, the body uses whatever substitute is available to build those cells, causing them to malfunction. DHA is sadly lacking in our modern diets, causing an epidemic of brain dysfunction, including depression, mood disorders, attention deficit disorder and a host of other medical problems. Similarly, a real egg contains ten times the vitamin E of a supermarket egg. To make matters worse, make-believe eggs are loaded with pesticides, hormones, antibiotics and a host of other toxins.

We have few real eggs because we have few real chickens. Real chickens must be raised outdoors in the fresh air and sunshine, eating their natural diet of bugs, worms, pigweed, dandelions and other living foods. Most of today's chickens are cage reared, confined in factories where they do not obtain the benefits of exercise or sunlight and are fed nutritionally deficient, processed chicken feed. Neither the meat nor the eggs of these unhealthy animals support healthy human life.

Commercial chickens are fed an incredibly deficient and toxic diet. They are so malnourished and unhealthy that they must be fed a lifetime of antibiotics and other drugs to keep them alive. Ninety percent of commercial chickens have cancer at the time of their slaughter. If these chickens' cells are so malnourished and unhealthy, how can you expect your cells to be healthy when you eat their meat and eggs?

Pork is no different. Pigs are fed a diet of recycled waste, filled with toxins, and more than 80 percent have pneumonia at their time of slaughter. Likewise with beef, cattle fattened in feed lots are so malnourished and sick that they require a variety of drugs just to keep them alive. In *Diet for a New America,* John Robbins described their typical diet:

[S]awdust laced with ammonia and feathers, shredded newspaper (complete with all the colors of toxic ink from the Sunday comics and advertising circulars), "plastic hay," processed sewage, inedible tallow and grease, poultry litter, cement dust, and cardboard scraps, not to mention the insecticides, antibiotics and hormones. Artificial flavors and aromas are added to trick the poor animals into eating this stuff.

The animals are not the only ones tricked. The consumer is "tricked" into buying these make-believe foods and into thinking that they contain the nutrients required to support healthy life. Dr. Joseph Beasley in *The Kellogg Report* wrote that shortchanging nutrients over a period of time "is bound to involve human illness, particularly chronic conditions such as today's high-technology medicine can't seem to get a handle on." Again and again, well-meaning parents go to the store thinking they are feeding their families fresh, wholesome foods, only to be fooled by the multitude of offerings of deficient, make-believe food products.

Carl Pfeiffer, Ph.D., M.D., related in *Mental and Elemental Nutrients* an experiment at the University of California, Irvine. Healthy rats were fed foods that an average American would purchase in a supermarket: white bread, sugar, eggs, milk, ground beef, cabbage, potatoes, tomatoes, oranges, apples, bananas and coffee. The rats developed a variety of diseases. Dr. Pfeiffer concluded that if the average human diet could not support the health of rats, then it probably would not do much better for humans.

In *Diet for a Poisoned Planet,* David Steinman describes an experiment in which four sets of rats were fed different diets. The first set ate natural foods and drank clean water. Throughout the three-month experiment, these rats remained alert, calm and social. The second set was fed the same food as the first, with the addition of hot dogs. These rats became

violent and fought each other aggressively. The third set ate
sugar-coated breakfast cereal and drank fruit punch. These rats
became nervous, hyperactive and aimless. The fourth set was
fed only sugar donuts and cola. These rats had trouble sleeping,
became extremely fearful and were unable to function as a
social unit. The poor nutrition of these foods (not to mention the
toxic food additives) had a profound effect on the behavior of
these animals. Many children today struggle with hyperactive,
antisocial and even violent behaviors. The time has come to
consider how their diet may be causing this behavior.

More Unreal Than Ever

As if our foods were not "make-believe" enough, modern
technology has taken another unhealthy leap. We now have
totally artificial, synthesized products that are consumed as
"food." The food industry is creating products such as artificial
sweeteners (saccharine and aspartame) and man-made fats,
including margarine, Olestra and nondairy creamer. As Paul
Stitt, author of *Fighting the Food Giants,* wrote, "An ever
increasing proportion of the food we eat is no longer even food
but is now a conglomerate of high-priced chemistry experiments designed to simulate food." More and more Americans
are eating these fabricated, imitation, processed foods; if you
want to eat a good diet, you cannot subsist on foods that are not
real—foods that are completely foreign to the body.

What are the real foods that your body needs in order to
become healthy and stay healthy? Your body needs nutrients:
vitamins, minerals, amino acids, essential oils, oxygen, water,
sunlight and fuel (calories). With the exception of water, air
and sunshine, the nutrients necessary to keep your cells
healthy must come primarily from the healthy plant and animal cells that you eat. If the fruits, vegetables, meats and other
foods that you eat are not healthy, they cannot keep you
healthy. If you are hoping for health, but eating a diet that is

made up of unhealthy plants and animals, or foods so highly processed that they no longer resemble plants or animals, you are hoping for the impossible.

A professor of chemistry wanted to demonstrate the superiority of fresh foods to his class. He purchased "fresh" oranges at a local supermarket and measured their vitamin C content. *There was none!* Unpleasantly surprised, he traced the oranges back to their source. He found they had been harvested while still green, stored for two years and then artificially colored prior to being sold as "fresh fruit." This is what the consumer is up against and why purchasing fresh, organic produce is so important.

One Size Does Not Fit All

The amount of nutrients required for optimal nutrition differs for every person and changes as a person's life progresses. We are not genetic cookie-cutter replicas of each other. In addition, individual factors can affect our nutritional needs, such as age, physical activity, climate, illness, injury, pregnancy or menstruation. Your need for calcium may be far higher than your neighbor's; your neighbor's requirements for vitamin C may differ widely from yours.

In his book *Nutrition Against Disease,* biochemist Roger Williams, Ph.D., reported on laboratory animals that were bred to have similar genes and, theoretically, have similar nutritional needs. Yet, some animals were found to need forty times as much vitamin A as others. Similarly, human nutritional requirements operate across a wide range. Williams described another study performed on healthy young men which demonstrated that their needs for calcium varied almost sixfold.

Does someone in your family catch colds and flus noticeably more often than everyone else? Have you considered that his or her need for vitamin C (vital for immune function) might be higher than everyone else's? Is vitamin C deficiency a problem for them, not because they get less of it, but because they need more? Researcher and Nobel laureate Linus Pauling was plagued with frequent colds and flu all of his adult life until he started taking high doses of vitamin C. Likewise, women have special nutritional needs (especially when pregnant or menstruating), as do elderly people, athletes and anyone who is fighting off an infection or suffering from a chronic disease. When it comes to nutritional needs, the "average person" does not exist.

Women are more likely to be nutritionally deficient than men. Why? Because women typically eat less food but still require roughly the same amount of nutrients. That women are more susceptible to certain diseases—including osteoporosis, chronic fatigue syndrome and autoimmune diseases—is no coincidence.

Because of reduced activity and appetite, older people require fewer calories (fuel), but they retain the same need for nutrients; in fact, nutritional needs may actually increase with aging (not to mention that digestion of food and assimilation of nutrients is often impaired in older people). Unfortunately, elderly people often are less able to buy and prepare fresh foods, and they often subsist on packaged, processed or frozen foods, thus consuming fewer nutrients. This diet makes a bad situation worse, contributing to widespread disease and disability among our older population.

Almost certainly, you have, for at least a few nutrients, unique needs that are substantially higher than average. More than a quarter century ago, medical pioneers like Dr. Carl Pfeiffer were able to use this concept to cure many cases of "incurable" schizophrenia by giving patients extra vitamins and minerals (above and beyond what was available through a regular diet). With their nutritional needs being met, Pfeiffer's schizophrenic patients were able to return to a completely normal life. Such nutrient deficiencies are a major cause of the many mental and behavioral problems in our society.

Arbitrary Standards

Although science has proved that we have individual nutritional needs, at present we have no way of measuring each person's needs. The Recommended Daily Allowances (or RDAs) that are listed on foods and vitamin supplements are arbitrary. They do not provide accurate information about what you need in order to stay healthy. These standards are a measurement only of the minimum dosage necessary to prevent a diagnosable deficiency disease, such as scurvy (a vitamin C deficiency disease common to sailors who went too long without fresh fruits and vegetables). You can easily meet RDA standards and still lack the nutrients necessary to prevent other diseases not specifically known as "deficiency diseases." In fact, optimal health usually requires at least several times the RDA values.

In reality, however, most people do not meet even these minimum standards. A study by Professor Suzanne Murphy at the University of California, Berkeley, published in the November 1992 issue of the *Journal of the American Dietetic Association,* measured the diets of 5,884 people for fifteen essential nutrients. The average person consistently measured below two-thirds of the RDAs for three to six essential nutrients. A separate study, sponsored by the U.S. Department of Agriculture, examined ten essential nutrients in the diets of 21,500 people. In that study, not a single person was obtaining 100 percent of the RDAs for all ten nutrients on a daily basis—not one person out of 21,500!

Virtually all Americans are chronically deficient in at least one and usually several nutrients, even when measured against the artificially low RDA standards. When we consider that good health requires several times the RDA, the true magnitude of the problem becomes apparent. That problem is compounded by the fact that nutrients must act as a team in order to keep you healthy.

Of the more than fifty known essential nutrients, each must

be available to the body on a daily basis and in the correct amounts and ratios to each other. Rather than acting by themselves, nutrients act in combination with each other; a shortage of even one starts a chain of events that can result in extensive nutritional deficiencies and body system malfunctions.

In *The Kellogg Report,* Dr. Joseph Beasley examines how one specific nutrient deficiency (vitamin B_3) has far-reaching ramifications: A vitamin B_3 deficiency impairs absorption of vitamin C, which impairs absorption of iron, which causes excessive copper absorption, which inhibits nickel metabolism, which in turn adversely affects iron metabolism, and on and on.

If all those can occur from a deficiency of just one nutrient (vitamin B_3 in this case), just imagine what happens in the bodies of most Americans, who are chronically deficient in several nutrients.

The most common deficiencies are calcium; zinc; magnesium; chromium; vitamins A, E, C and B_6; and folic acid. What you must recognize is that you cannot miss even one member of the nutrition package and hope to be healthy. The way to assure you are getting what you need is to eat a wide range of real foods that are rich in nutrition, keep the Big Four and other "make-believe" foods out of your diet, and take high-quality nutritional supplements.

A Diet That Really Works

As a child growing up in a Boston suburb, I remember food shopping with my mother at several farms in our town. The farmers maintained the mineral content of their soils with traditional methods of crop rotation, mulch and manure. All through the summer and even into the fall, those farms supplied our town with freshly harvested, organically grown, fully ripened fruits and vegetables. Everybody in town could share in the nutrition those small local farms provided. By the late 1950s, all the farms had been sold for housing develop-ments, as happened to many small farms across the United States. From a real estate standpoint, subdivisions may be the best use of the land, but from a health standpoint, development is a disaster. Lost with those local farms was the superior nutrition contained within fresh, organically produced foods. What has replaced them are commercially produced, toxic, nutritionally deficient supermarket foods.

Our biological ancestors ate living food directly as nature provided—often with no alternative. If you were hungry and found a berry bush, fresh berries were what you ate. Likewise, a hunter might eat an animal right after the kill, its flesh still containing living cells filled with vital nutrients. Nature works that way. Within these hunting and gathering parameters we evolved biologically; even today our nutritional needs are best served with living foods that are as unchanged as possible from the way nature provides them. Instead, we often settle for food in very different forms: cooked, dehydrated, ground, canned, frozen, hydrolyzed, hydrogenated, irradiated or other-wise modified. By eating a diet that consists primarily of these "altered" foods, we run the risk of being deficient in fundamental nutrients that are contained only within the whole, intact, living cells of other organisms.

Your body needs to burn calories every day to provide energy. Although Americans are seldom deficient in calories, almost always they are deficient in nutrients. *We must learn to count nutrients, not calories.* Your body builds more than ten million new cells every second. If the foods you eat do not contain sufficient nutrients needed to build and maintain those cells, an "eat more" message is sent to the brain. This happens regardless of how many calories are in your diet. A body that is starving for nutrients seeks out more food, and weight gain likely results. Eating just one hundred calories more than you burn, on a daily basis, translates to roughly twelve pounds of added fat per year. Try that ten years in a row!

Many Americans are both malnourished and overweight. Obesity is a major health problem in America today, regardless of age or economic status. According to recent government statistics, 63 percent of American adults are overweight. When you eat real, nutritious foods (typically lower in calories), your body obtains the nutrients it needs and you likely do not have intense food cravings. If a large part of your diet is made up of real foods, becoming overweight is difficult.

Unfortunately, overweight people (or those wishing to avoid becoming overweight) often cut down on their overall food (calories) intake, without making changes in what types of foods they eat. This results in more malnourishment and stronger food cravings. Consuming 2,000 calories yet obtaining little or no nutrition is frightfully easy: a small candy bar (280 calories and almost no nutrition), two soft drinks (600 calories and no nutrition), and a hamburger/fries/shake meal (1,180 calories and only a little nutrition). This intake totals 2,060 calories yet offers a serious case of malnutrition. That diet provides some protein, carbohydrate and fat that the body can use—but is seriously lacking in vitamins, minerals, phytonutrients, enzymes, fiber, essential fatty acids and other nutrients necessary to construct healthy cells and maintain good health. Lacking these nutrients, the body must deplete its nutrient reserves in order to keep functioning. When the reserves run out, cells suffer from deficiency, and they cease to self-regulate and self-repair. Disease follows. Meanwhile, you are still hungry and adding more weight because your body is short of nutrients.

Magic Capsules

How do real foods support the health and function of your cells whereas processed foods do not? Here's one example: Whole grains (such as wheat, oats, millet and quinoa) are seeds that contain all the ingredients necessary to create a new plant—to create a new life. They are like magic capsules. The nutrients in these capsules that are necessary to create life are also necessary to sustain your life. However, as soon as this life-creating capsule has been opened (due to cutting, mashing or grinding), oxygen reacts with the chemicals inside, causing the nutrients to deteriorate. At this point, the seed can no longer produce a new life, nor can it sustain yours as well as before. Our ancestors did not have such nutrient losses in their grains, which were eaten whole or coarsely ground, rather than processed into nutritionally worthless white flour. Remember the Hunzas? They coarsely ground grains and immediately made nutritious flat breads, minimizing nutrient loss.

Foods that are nutritious but nontoxic come from the following categories:

- *Organic foods* produced naturally without any man-made chemicals, such as pesticides, herbicides, fertilizers, preservatives, antibiotics, hormones, processed animal feed, etc. These foods are generally higher in nutrients and lower in toxins than nonorganic (commercially produced) foods of the same type.

- *Fresh foods* harvested at their peak of nutrition (ripeness) and consumed shortly thereafter. Food that is harvested does not gain any more nutrition (even though it may continue to ripen), and in fact, nutrition begins to decline. Some foods deteriorate more quickly than others, but the point is that you want to eat your food as soon after harvesting as possible. The more the food sits around (during harvesting, storage, transportation and distribution), the more nutrition it will lose.

- *Unprocessed foods,* minimally altered from the way that nature provides. Avoid foods that are cooked, peeled, cut, ground, dehydrated, frozen, canned, etc. Unprocessed foods are whole, complete foods, rather than just part of a food (whole grains instead of flour made from grains, for example, or potatoes with the peel still on).

Because we cannot all revert to hunting, gathering, growing our own food and eating it fresh and raw, we must learn to evaluate the foods that are available to us and make choices that are both healthy and realistic. We must take the "black and white" nutritional knowledge outlined above and apply it to our lives in the best shade of gray that we can.

Poisoned in the Nursery

Much of the nutrition trouble we face begins before food leaves commercial farms. Modern agricultural practices and chemicals (such as chemical fertilizers, insecticides, herbicides and fungicides) produce ever-increasing quantities of food, but the chemicals reduce the nutritional quality of the food and deplete the soil of nutrients needed to produce future quality crops.

Chemical fertilizers, which are supposed to put nutrients into the soil, actually end up causing nutrients to be removed from the soil. The most common chemical fertilizers, which support high food production, add three major nutrients to the soil: nitrogen, phosphorous and potassium. But the plants require many other nutrients absorbed from the soil, such as zinc, calcium, magnesium, selenium, germanium, chromium, manganese, nickel and molybdenum. Chemical fertilizers do not supply these nutrients. By not replacing these nutrients and by growing more food on the same land year after year after year, critical nutrients continually are lost from the soil, leading to nutrient-deficient soil, nutrient-deficient crops, nutrient-deficient farm animals and nutrient-deficient human beings.

In her 1976 book *The Living Soil,* Lady Eve Balfour describes an eighteen-year experiment on three farms with similar soil profiles. One of the farms was managed organically, one chemically, and the third, a mixture of the two. During this eighteen-year study, the soil on the organic farm was found to have the highest mineral content. Not coincidentally, the dairy herd on that farm was healthier, produced more milk and had higher reproductive capacity.

The use of chemical fertilizers triggers a series of problems as plants struggle to cope with deficient soils and toxic attacks. Plants grown in nutrient-deficient soils are less healthy and more vulnerable to insects, molds, fungi, viruses, bacteria and weeds. The susceptibility leads to the use of other agricultural chemicals, such as pesticides, herbicides and fungicides, to protect sick plants. These toxic chemicals create "dead soils," killing not only the undesirable organisms but also the helpful organisms (earthworms, insects, bacteria and fungi) that are responsible for taking minerals out of the soil and converting them into forms that plants can use. When these bacteria and fungi are killed, the plants no longer receive adequate nutrition.

Insecticides, fungicides and herbicides accumulate in the soil to a level where they inhibit plant growth. These poor growing conditions have spurred the development of new kinds of plants, such as hybrid and genetically modified crops. In creating genetically modified plants, which humankind has never eaten before, we may have (unknowingly) altered the nutritional value of the plants, as well as made them more toxic or allergenic. More and more genetically modified foods are contaminating the food supply with novel and unnatural varieties of organisms. (See chapter 9 for more information.)

Shelves Stocked with Old Food

I can remember, as a child on my uncle's farm, picking ripe apples from the trees and eating them then and there. I can remember harvesting fresh peas, strawberries and sweet corn from our own garden and eating them raw within minutes of harvesting. Not only do fresh foods taste better; they are substantially better for health. Much of the food purchased in a standard supermarket today is old. Presumably fresh produce such as apples, oranges and cucumbers are put in cold storage and can be anywhere from months to years old. Supermarket eggs are commonly anywhere from six weeks to six months old, and they still can be labeled as "fresh."

Food is reasonably hardy, but nutrients are not. Nutrients are quite fragile and are destroyed by heat, light, oxygen and overly long storage. The most fragile vitamins are C, B_1 and B_5. Unless you grow food yourself or obtain it freshly harvested from a local farmer, it's likely the food does not have the nutrition you think it has.

Irradiated foods may be years old before you eat them and thus completely devoid of vitamins. Fruits and vegetables undergo substantial destruction of nutrients in modern cold storage. In *The Kellogg Report,* Dr. Joseph Beasley offered examples of the nutritional loss that occurs after harvesting:

- Spinach and asparagus lose 50 to 70 percent of their folic acid when kept at room temperature for three days.
- Vegetables such as asparagus, broccoli and green beans typically lose 50 percent of their vitamin C before they reach the produce counter.
- Potatoes lose as much as 78 percent of their vitamin C during long-term storage at 36°F.
- Blanching of vegetables prior to freezing can destroy up to half of the vitamins.
- Freezing meat can destroy up to 70 percent of its vitamins.

Commercial, make-believe foods lack nutrients not only because of losses after harvest, but also because food is frequently harvested before it is ripe. This practice may be necessary for our modern distribution system (to bring food to the consumer before it rots), but early harvesting also reduces nutrition. The ripening process is critical to develop the full vitamin and mineral content of a food; vitamin and mineral content rise near the peak of ripeness. Also, flavor improves.

The carrots you buy in the supermarket may look ripe, but they frequently turn that bright orange (ripe) color during transit through the distribution system. If they are not ripened while still in the soil (and most are not), they will lack essential nutrients. Vine-ripened, freshly harvested tomatoes are loaded with vitamins, minerals and phytonutrients (natural chemicals in plants that benefit our health)—unlike commercial tomatoes that are picked green and artificially ripened with ethylene gas. Naturally ripened tomatoes were found to contain one-third more vitamin C than those harvested green and immature. Foods harvested before they are ripe never develop certain nutrients at all. Certain phytonutrients (substances found in ripe tomatoes known to help prevent diseases such as cataracts, macular degeneration and even cancer) are lacking in the typical supermarket tomato because these substances develop in the last stages of ripening.

While having all kinds of food available to us all year round is wonderful, we pay the price with our health because the food must often be harvested before it is ripe, transported long distances, stored for long periods and artificially ripened. Even though such foods may look and taste fine, they are substantially less nutritious. They are "make-believe" foods.

Beware of Food Guillotines

Even foods that are truly fresh and ripe can nevertheless be nutritionally destroyed if you prepare them improperly. Our biological ancestors usually did not cook or process their foods. Foods were eaten fresh and raw. The healthy Hunzas ate 80 percent of their diet raw. Their foods not only had more nutrition to begin with (because of traditional farming techniques and rich soils), they also did not typically diminish that nutrition by cooking. Nobel laureate Linus Pauling believed that the mostly raw, mostly vegetarian, unprocessed diet of our biological ancestors provided a level of nutritional quality far superior to the food supply available today.

The bulk of the modern American diet comes from processed foods that have been deliberately altered from the way
nature provided. This altering includes trimming, peeling,
chopping, blending, mashing, commercial refining and cooking. While some degree of processing may be necessary, there
are many degrees of processing, from the simple slicing of a
carrot for your salad all the way to the grinding and bleaching
of wheat in order to make white flour. The most significant
causes of malnutrition, other than commercial farming and
distribution techniques, are cooking and processing.

In general, proteins in food are the most stable (less damaged by processing), while vitamins are the most easily damaged. A cucumber loses a quarter of its vitamin C just by
slicing it to make a salad. If the salad stands around for an
hour, the loss goes up to a third, and if it stands for three hours,
half its vitamin C will be gone. Fresh orange juice loses
almost a fifth of its vitamin B_1 within twenty-four hours, even
when refrigerated. Cooking and mashing a potato will diminish vitamin C by 80 percent.

The heat used in cooking foods damages nutrients and typically makes them more difficult to digest. Cooking even damages protein (the most hardy of nutrients). Consider oatmeal:
In the *Food and Nutrition Encyclopedia,* Aubrey Ensminger
reported that dry oatmeal contains 14 percent protein, but that
figure drops to only 2 percent after it is cooked—a loss of 85
percent. Cooking common vegetables, such as carrots, can
cause losses of 75 percent of the vitamin C, 70 percent of the
vitamin B_1, 50 percent of the vitamin B_2 and 60 percent of
vitamin B_3. *The higher the heat and the longer the cooking
time, the more nutrients your food loses.*

Heating food deactivates its enzymes (the cellular machinery that manufactures all the products our cells make).
Although the human body is capable of making its own
enzymes, we also receive enzymes directly from our food.

Cooking destroys these enzymes. Eating cooked foods stresses the body, which must manufacture extra enzymes in order to digest food and compensate for enzymes lost in cooked food. By eating cooked foods, you can actually lose more nutrients than you gain. Consuming sufficient enzymes is one reason that eating raw foods is so important. Cooked foods contribute to our epidemic of chronic disease.

Although the health benefits of raw foods need emphasis, a few words of caution are important about raw animal products (such as eggs, meat, fish and poultry). Even though nature intended us to eat raw foods—animal products included—today's hazards of bacterial, viral and parasitic infections make raw animal foods dangerous. Also, raw animal foods must not touch other foods intended to be eaten raw.

Even just a few generations ago, people typically ate more raw food than they do now, and the trend toward cooked and processed foods appears to be worsening. According to U.S. Department of Agriculture statistics, over the last century average consumption of fresh apples declined by more than three-fourths, fresh cabbage by more than two-thirds and fresh fruit by more than one-third. During that same period, consumption of processed vegetables went up hundreds of percent and consumption of processed fruits went up by about 1,000 percent. *Eating processed fruits and vegetables (canned, dried, frozen, etc.) is fundamentally inferior to eating fresh fruits and vegetables.*

Eat for Your Future, Too

The nutritionally deprived, cooked and processed foods you eat today will damage your health tomorrow, as well as the health of your unborn children and grandchildren in the years to come.

This profound concept was demonstrated in the 1940s by Francis Pottenger Jr., M.D., and published in his book

Pottenger's Cats. More than nine hundred cats, some fed a diet of raw food and some a cooked-food diet, showed striking differences in their own health as well as the health of their offspring. Within six months, the cats eating the cooked food developed numerous health problems. Subsequent generations suffered infections, dental problems, vision problems, skin problems, allergies, arthritis, miscarriages and behavioral changes—including nervousness, viciousness and violent behavior. Each new generation was sicker than the last. By the third generation, almost all the cats suffered from allergies and had trouble reproducing because of miscarriages and still-births. Meanwhile, the cats on the raw-food diet remained healthy and well-behaved, generation after generation. We have much to learn from Pottenger's work; the most significant (and ominous) implication is the impact of poor nutrition, supplied by cooked food, on the health of future generations.

Another case dramatically proves the need for raw, fresh foods. During World War I, sailors aboard a German cruiser, *Kronprinz Wilhelm,* ate beef, ham, bacon, cheese, potatoes, canned vegetables, dried peas/beans, white bread, margarine, tea, coffee, sugar, condensed milk, cake, champagne and beer. Their entire diet consisted of cooked and processed foods. After six months on this diet, the crew was experiencing shortness of breath, paralysis, atrophied muscles, enlarged hearts, constipation, anemia, and muscle and joint pain. Fifty men could no longer stand. After eight months, 500 were sick, 110 were bedridden, and they were falling at a rate of four per day. New symptoms included pleurisy, rheumatism, pneumonia and other infections, and fractures and wounds that would not heal.

An emergency stop in Virginia brought a new diet containing some raw fruits and vegetables. After ten days, the men stopped falling sick; forty-seven had been discharged. Conditions gradually improved thereafter. Access to fresh, raw food was all it took. Notably, the only people on the ship who did not get sick were the officers who had ongoing (if limited) access to raw fruits and vegetables, apparently providing just enough nutrition to make the difference between health and disease.

Think of all the people that you know who suffer from allergies, gum disease, heart problems, vision problems, arthritis, antisocial behavior, miscarriages and other health problems. Could malnutrition, perhaps even the malnutrition of their parents or grandparents before them, be contributing to their problems? Talk to those people you know who have lived in good health into their eighties, nineties or even older. Chances are they grew up on farms and ate plenty of raw, real food during their developmental years. By contrast, consider the deteriorating health of many people in the baby boomer generation—the first humans to develop eating processed, "TV dinner" diets starting in the 1950s.

Families today often have grandparents that lived (or are still living) into their nineties, while the next generation is getting sick and dying in their seventies or sixties. Today's young people are plagued with problems such as cancer, asthma, diabetes, allergies, obesity, poor eyesight, dyslexia, birth defects and other problems, and are likely to die at even younger ages. An epidemic of allergic disease is occurring in industrialized countries, especially in people born after 1960. The prevalence of asthma has quadrupled over the last two decades. Could something as simple as nutritional deficiency be a major contributor to violent behavior and vicious crimes? Many reasons exist to believe so. Many of our young people can no longer reproduce; some estimates are as high as one in five. These problems were rare just a few generations ago when our grandparents and great-grandparents were eating more organic, fresh, and unprocessed raw foods. These problems did not exist among well-nourished populations such as the Hunzas.

How You Eat Matters

Millions of Americans are plagued with heartburn, abdominal pain, bloating, gas, nausea, bowel difficulties and other digestive problems. Much more than inconvenient, these are telltale signs of poor digestion—resulting in deficiency and toxicity, i.e., disease. To eliminate these problems, follow a few simple guidelines, which will support healthy digestion. You can choose digestion habits that will bring nutrients into your cells and let wastes out of your body efficiently.

The basic steps of good digestion are as follows: First, eat the right combinations of foods, because certain foods digest better together than others. Next, chew your food well, to assist in the digestive process. Nutrients must be absorbed properly through your intestinal walls and transported throughout your body to all the cells that need them. Finally, wastes must excrete from the body. Any interference with any of these steps of the digestive process can cause both deficiency and toxicity. Deficiency may occur if food is not properly digested and absorbed. Toxicity occurs when undigested food "sits" too long, either in the stomach or in the intestines, where it rots, ferments and putrefies, creating toxins.

Although eating a variety of foods is a great idea, we are not designed to digest them all at the same time. Learning which foods go well with each other is what "food combining" is all about. Our digestive systems have adapted and evolved over many thousands of years; until recently humankind did not eat the combinations of foods that are now "normal" to us. Our hunter-gatherer ancestors often ate foods directly from their source, usually one at a time because there was no way to preserve or store them. Our ancestors certainly did not cook up three- or four-course meals that combine all sorts of different proteins, starches, sugars, fruits and vegetables.

When we are young, our digestive systems are working at

peak performance and indulging in digestive indiscretions may be possible. As we age, digestive capacity diminishes. Forcing the body to digest incompatible foods results in improperly digested food that produces dangerous toxins. Also, undigested food deprives us of essential nutrients.

Food combining principles are important because each food category has different digestive requirements. The requirements for proteins and starches are radically different; if you eat them both at the same time you cannot digest either one well. Proteins digest in an acid environment, whereas starches digest in an alkaline environment. Your digestive system has the ability to create either environment, but cannot create both at the same time. Instead, combine proteins or starches with vegetables, which are highly nutritious and combine well with either one.

Fruit has special digestive requirements and should be eaten alone. Fruit is easy to digest and is meant to pass through the digestive system quickly. If not, such as when combined with protein or starch, the fruit sugar ferments in the stomach, often manifested by bloating and gas. If sweet and acid fruits are to be eaten together, eat the acid fruits first. Melons should be eaten alone or combined with other melons because they take even less time to digest than other fruits and should pass quickly through your digestive system in order to prevent sugar fermentation.

To learn about food combinations that work well together and those that do not, consider a few simple food categories: proteins, starches, vegetables, and three kinds of fruits (sweet, acid and melons). Remember these simple rules:

Vegetables with proteins, okay.
Vegetables with starches, okay.
No protein with starch (avoid meat and potatoes, spaghetti and meatballs, fish and rice, etc.).

Eat fruit alone. (Acid fruits with nuts and seeds, okay.
Acid fruits with sweet fruits, okay, although acid fruits
should be consumed first. Eat melons alone, except with
other melons.)

Not certain which of your favorite foods fall into which
categories? Here are examples:

Protein	Eggs, meat, fish, fowl, nuts, seeds, avocado, coconut, sprouts, milk products.
Starch	Corn, wheat, barley, rice, buckwheat, millet, oats, dried peas and beans, potatoes, yams, squash, flour (pasta/bread/pastries), sugar (candy/soft drinks/etc.).
Vegetables	Asparagus, tomatoes, okra, green beans, green peas, broccoli, bell peppers, brussels sprouts, cabbage, lettuce, celery, cucumber, beets, eggplant, spinach, mushrooms, zucchini, radish, artichoke, beets, carrots, cauliflower, chives, ginger, garlic, leeks, onion, shallots, scallions.
Sweet Fruits	Bananas, currants, figs, dates, raisins, prunes, dried fruits, grapes.
Acid Fruits	Lemons, oranges, grapefruits, other citrus fruits, kiwi, plum, pineapple, mango, papaya, all berries, nectarines, apples, cherries, pears, apricots, peaches.
Melons	Cantaloupe, casaba, crenshaw, honeydew, banana melon, watermelon.

Many of our traditional meals are comprised of wrong combinations. What we think of as a "good meal" is typically a
harmful combination of starch and protein—meat and potatoes, a burger and fries or a cheese pizza. We make the problem worse by accompanying meals with sugary drinks and
desserts; these combinations cause the food to ferment and

putrefy in the digestive system (and the protein/sugar combination also results in the formation of harmful AGEs—as described in the sugar section of the Big Four).

Learning how to apply proper food combinations to your diet can help your health, as it did for Andrea. Her high-profile career was interrupted when chronic fatigue and an autoimmune syndrome called lupus overwhelmed her. Before she came to see me, Andrea had been sick for five years and had exhausted all the remedies that modern medicine had to offer—with no help.

I encouraged Andrea to keep a food diary so that we could track what she was eating. The diary revealed that Andrea's diet consisted of a lot of processed junk ("make-believe" food). I taught her how to shop for "real" food and suggested special vitamin supplements. Within one week this woman—who had been chronically ill for five years—was starting to feel much better. She gained more energy and more mental clarity, and she began to have hope. Then she reached a plateau and seemed unable to make further improvement.

I suggested that Andrea prepare another food diary, this time looking at the combinations of foods she was eating. We found out why her recovery process stalled. Andrea's meal choices were causing maldigestion and creating toxins that were inhibiting her recovery. For example, she had gone out to a Sunday brunch and ate a breakfast consisting of a vegetable omelet (protein and vegetables, okay), hash-brown potatoes (starch with protein, not okay), toast with jelly (starch and sugar with protein, not okay), and a fruit cup (fruit with other foods, not okay). Combining egg protein with the starch of bread and potatoes was bad enough; the fermentation caused by combining that with sugar from fresh fruit and jelly made things worse.

By maldigesting her food, this meal was not supplying Andrea with the nutrition she thought she was consuming. At the same time her choices were creating toxins that were poisoning every cell in her body—certainly not what she had in mind when she ordered brunch. At another meal, Andrea had a sandwich made of organic, whole-wheat bread, organic turkey and organic lettuce. While definitely better than the breakfast, combining starch (bread) with protein (turkey) just does not work. I knew how important it would be for her health if she had a good understanding of basic food-combining rules. I taught her the simple rules of food combining: *vegetables with protein, okay; vegetables with starch, okay; no protein with starch; eat fruit alone.*

Andrea put these simple rules to work. Her health continued to improve, and she went into complete remission of all her chronic health problems—something she had been unable to do even with good food and supplements alone. Proper food combining was critical to this woman's wellness process, which is no surprise, because improper food combining causes disease.

It's All in the Technique

When you eat cooked foods, eating something raw first is best. Cooked food appears to be so alien to the human system that it can provoke an immune response, as if you are being exposed to a virus. Scientist Udo Erasmus, author of *Fats and Oils,* wrote:

> [W]hen cooked (or dead) food is eaten, a defense reaction occurs in the tissues of the stomach and digestive tract. This reaction is similar to the reaction we find in infections and around tumors and involves the accumulation of white blood cells, swelling, and a fever-like increase in temperature of the stomach and intestinal tissues. [As a result, we] experience tiredness after the meal. The same reaction takes place when half the food is eaten raw, but the cooked part is eaten first. When the

raw part of the food is eaten first, however, this reaction does not take place.

Chewing your food also is important. The style that many people use is "chomp, chomp, gulp—down the hatch!" Lack of proper chewing can cause maldigestion and contribute to disease. Many of our modern foods are easy to gulp down, requiring little help from the teeth (because of excessive cooking, processing and fat content). By contrast, real foods (whole foods and especially raw foods) tend to have more texture and fiber, and require more chewing. If you want good nutrition to support good health, you need to eat real food and you need to chew it well.

First, your teeth physically mash food into small particles. Then, your saliva combines enzymes with food as it is being chewed and helps to break down and digest it. The purpose of chewing is not simply to break the food into small enough chunks to swallow, although many people eat this way. The purpose of chewing is to assist the digestive process by grinding your food into small particles and coating them thoroughly with the digestive enzymes in your saliva.

There is an old saying: "Drink what you eat and eat what you drink." Solid food should be chewed thoroughly enough that it becomes liquid before you swallow it; liquid foods (such as juices and soups) should be "chewed" so that the enzymes in your saliva have time to work on them. Nutrition starts in your mind and in your mouth. Eat your food with the intent to nourish your body, rather than merely to fill the void in your stomach.

Rethink "Acid Indigestion"

After leaving the mouth, the chewed, enzyme-coated food moves to the stomach and triggers the release of hydrochloric acid and other digestive chemicals that further break down the food before it moves into the small intestine. In fact, until sufficient hydrochloric acid is present and food breakdown takes place, food does not leave the stomach. If undigested food sits in the stomach too long, it forms toxins and poisons you. Adequate hydrochloric acid is critical in the digestive process.

People often think that indigestion is caused by "too much acid"—commonly called "acid indigestion." While in some rare cases this diagnosis is valid, the overwhelming majority of acid symptoms originate from the opposite problem—too little hydrochloric acid. As a result, the food does not digest properly and remains in the stomach too long, whereupon the food rots and becomes acidic. Rotting food, not excessive digestive acids, causes an acid burn feeling. *Deliberately taking antacid tablets before you eat, to prevent acid indigestion, is not a good idea.* It only makes a bad situation worse. The best remedies for acid indigestion are to pay attention to basic food combining principles and to chew your food well. Supplementing with digestive enzymes also can be helpful. (Note: Supplementing with hydrochloric acid tablets is also possible, but this much more aggressive measure requires education and careful monitoring.)

Most absorption of nutrients takes place in the small intestine. By the time it reaches the small intestine, food must have undergone proper digestion. The small intestine extracts nutrients from the food and they enter the bloodstream. Waste products move along to the large intestine where they are excreted from the body.

Food not properly processed by the time it reaches the small intestine creates a host of problems. Poorly digested, putrefying, fermenting and rotting food particles in the intestines create vast amounts of toxins. Undigested food molecules can pass through the intestinal walls and move directly into the bloodstream. In the bloodstream the body recognizes these food molecules as foreign. The immune system may attack them. This response resembles a classic food allergy; poor digestion of a food can cause you to become allergic to it. Worse, each allergic reaction damages the intestinal tissue and makes it more permeable, perpetuating the problem. An increasing number of food allergies and numerous other health problems may result. These ongoing allergic reactions can overtax and exhaust the immune system, making you vulnerable to low-grade, chronic infections, such as chronic sinus infections.

Provided the digestive process goes well in the intestines, allowing the proper nutrients to enter the bloodstream, those nutrients must still go to the proper cells and then inside those cells. This activity often requires separate "transporter nutrients" (certain amino acids, for example) that also come from your diet. In other words, nutrients are used for many purposes, including delivery of other nutrients. This is one example of how nutrients work together in tandem, and why you cannot afford to miss a single one. Once the necessary nutrients have arrived at the target cells, they still need to pass through the cell membranes. If the membrane is not constructed properly (as described in the fats and oils section of the Big Four), new problems arise. Nutrients can have a difficult time being transported through cell membranes constructed from "bad" fats and oils (hydrogenated oils, refined supermarket oils, deep-fried foods and excessive saturated fats).

The final step in proper digestion is the elimination of waste products, which must be eliminated as quickly and efficiently as possible. Otherwise, toxins may reabsorb back into the body. The best ways to improve bowel function are to eat sufficient fiber, follow proper food combining and chew food well. If you select a food with good fiber content and then cook it, however, you may be short-changing yourself. Some of the fibrous structure of food can be lost in the cooking process, so be sure not to overcook.

Many people find it uncomfortable, even embarrassing, to

talk about their body's waste products. Being comfortable with these natural processes is important because one of the simplest ways to measure the health of your digestive system is to be aware of your bowel movements and to note the quality of your stools, in terms of frequency, texture and odor.

Most Americans are constipated; many have a bowel movement only every other day or think that one movement per day is ideal. Not true. If you do not have frequent, efficient elimination, then food wastes remain in your intestines, where they putrefy and poison you. Optimal is two or three bowel movements a day—one, at the very least. Loose stools or exceptionally dense stools are reflections of serious problems, especially if they persist. Well-formed and floating is a good rule of thumb. Excessive gases (stomach or intestinal) or stool odor also may indicate digestive trouble. Be aware of your elimination process, and if you have a problem, take steps to remedy it by following the guidelines in this chapter.

Choosing the Right Dietary Supplements

Eating good foods and digesting them well may not be sufficient to make sure your cells receive all the nutrients they need every day. Supplementing your diet with high-quality vitamin, mineral and essential fatty acid supplements is also important.

Supplements have become a necessity in our society for two reasons: First, the supply of nutrients is down. Intensive commercial farming, depleted soils and food processing have reduced the nutritional content of our food so dramatically that our diets no longer contain the nutrients required by our cells to maintain good health. Second, our need for certain nutrients is up because of the effects of environmental pollution, which puts extra stress on the body. Responding to this stress uses up essential nutrients, in particular antioxidants, such as vitamins A, C and E. With the supply of nutrients down and the need for nutrients up, is it any wonder that three out of four Americans have a diagnosable chronic disease? Supplementation is necessary to bridge the gap between what we need and what comes from our diet.

Most physicians (who, on average, receive only two and a half hours of nutritional training during four years of medical school) often tell you that supplements are not necessary—that they make little more than expensive urine. The position often taken by physicians is that you can get all the nutrition you need to maintain health by eating a balanced diet of commercially produced foods. You know by now that this claim is absolutely false.

Numerous studies have shown that virtually all Americans are not receiving the recommended amounts of nutrients on a daily basis. Many nutritional researchers (myself included) believe that, in our modern world, obtaining the nutrients we need from diet alone, even if we eat good foods, is impossible. Over the last quarter century, research has established that a huge gap exists between the small amounts of nutrients required for preventing overt nutritional-deficiency diseases and the large amounts of nutrients required to maintain optimal health and fortify our bodies against disease in general. Dietary supplements help fill the gaps in your nutrition, especially in those nutrients for which you, as an individual, may have a particularly high need. One final note: Supplements are not an invitation to eat a poor diet; they are to be used in addition to healthy foods.

Countless people have been cured of chronic health problems by the addition of dietary supplements. Consider Albert, a man who sought my advice several years ago. Albert had been suffering from serious, "untreatable" depression for almost a decade. He had exhausted his resources going to hospitals, clinics and physicians, but nothing had helped. His life was a living hell, and he was suicidal.

At our first meeting I learned that he subsisted on a meager diet consisting mostly of processed foods and that he was addicted to sugar. I suggested that he eliminate sugar and incorporate fresh, raw fruits and vegetables into his diet. I recommended a supplement program of specific vitamins and essential fatty acids. Albert was skeptical that these seemingly simple suggestions would make any real difference, considering how many "expert doctors" he had already seen. In less than a week after starting the diet and supplement program, Albert called to say that he felt as if a great burden had been lifted from him. He was no longer feeling suicidal. In all of his years of treatment for clinical depression, I was the first person who had suggested that poor nutrition could be the cause. In fact, poor nutrition is the leading cause of depression (and almost every other disease).

Although Albert had been taking nutritional supplements before he saw me, he had been taking the wrong kinds of supplements (those with low bioactivity, which means they were in a form that the body could not easily absorb or use). Ultimately, bioactivity is critical to whether supplements will be effective or not. When institutions like the Centers for Disease and Control and Prevention and the National Academy of Sciences have performed large-scale population studies to measure the benefits of taking supplements, they have failed to find any benefits because most people are taking poor-quality supplements.

Quality is everything—in supplements, as well as food. For Albert, quality supplements (with high bioactivity at the cellular level) made all the difference. Having been a technical consultant to vitamin companies, I can tell you that of all the vitamin products on the market today, few actually do much good.

An investigative report aired on NBC's *Today* show in 1990 determined that 36 percent of the multivitamin brands tested did not dissolve soon enough to be absorbed and be of use to the body. In fact, some never dissolved at all! These failures included only the most popular brands. The numbers of failing brands would have been far higher had all the minor brands been measured. NBC's testing also allowed a generous one-hour for the pills to dissolve. Using a more conservative (and appropriate) time of forty-five minutes would have made almost half the tested brands fail. *Almost half of all vitamin brands are not going to do your body any good, yet these are what most people use.* One reason that these brands fail is because they are filled with additives, which can constitute up to half of the volume of the pill. These additives are used as fillers, binders, lubricants, colors and preservatives, but they can cause real problems—not only interfering with the pills' ability to dissolve and with nutrient absorption, but also introducing many harmful contaminants and allergens into your body.

Most vitamins marketed today are synthetics and often contain petroleum residues from their manufacture. Some of these synthetic molecules are fundamentally different from natural vitamins, which affects the ability of your body to utilize them. For example, synthetic vitamin E is far less biologically active than vitamin E derived from natural sources. Synthetic beta-carotene actually can cause a deficiency of other carotenes.

Nutritional supplements are available at different levels of quality and price because of the variety of manufacturing processes used to create them. Each brand exhibits different properties and bioactivities. Trying to select a vitamin brand can be a bewildering experience. I found that comparing two different brands with exactly the same list of ingredients was not even possible, because how these ingredients are made is just as important as what is printed on the label. Unless you are a chemist or you know exactly how the supplement was made (and how the body metabolizes nutrients), distinguishing the difference between two seemingly identical products is almost impossible. The initial quality, chemical form, age of the ingredients, how they were handled (whether or not they were exposed to moisture, heat, light and oxygen during their storage or manufacture), and what other chemicals they are combined with in the formula has everything to do with the bioactivity of the final supplement.

When I was recovering from my chemical hypersensitivity, I was unable to take most vitamins because of their chemical contaminants. Vitamin supplements were critically important in my recovery process, but first I had to find pills that were pure, biologically active and uncontaminated. The contaminants in most pills (that were making me sick) also tax the health of people who are healthy, even if they are not aware of it.

Seeking manufacturers who use quality ingredients along with good manufacturing practices is vitally important. Most of the supplements on the market today are not worthwhile, as many do not contain what is professed on the labels, and many are even toxic—contaminated by substances such as heavy metals, solvent residues, pesticides, artificial colors and allergens. The supplement market is unregulated; you simply cannot trust vitamin pills unless you know how they are made. Even the best-selling brands of vitamins are not something I would take myself or recommend to others.

Although you cannot always trust labels, I have developed some convenient rules of thumb that help me to quickly evaluate the quality of vitamin supplements. First, check to see if cheap ingredients can be recognized on the label. Cheap ingredients usually suggest that the remainder of the product is not of high quality. Does cost matter? Yes, because it costs more to purchase pure ingredients that are in the more bioactive forms. For example, calcium carbonate is an ingredient used in many mineral formulas, supposedly to supply calcium, and it does to a certain degree, but very inefficiently. Compounds such as calcium citrate, calcium fumarate, or calcium malate are far more biologically active and are much better choices. However, they are much more expensive. The uneducated consumer seeking a calcium supplement will usually choose a formula based on price or appearance or how much calcium it contains rather than chemical composition and bioactivity.

Paying attention to the chemical composition of the nutrients is more important. Some chemical forms are better than others because of their superior bioavailability. The poor ones should be avoided. Below are some guidelines for choosing the quality of mineral supplements:

Poor Bioactivity	Acceptable Bioactivity	Optimal Bioactivity
Carbonate	Aminoate	Ascorbate
(e.g., calcium carbonate)	Chelate	Citrate
Oxide	Gluconate	Fumarate
(e.g., magnesium oxide)		Malate
Sulfate		Picolinate
Phosphate		Succinate
		Tartrate

Now look at the vitamins. The easiest way is to check the B vitamins, specifically vitamins B_2 and B_6. In a high-quality formula, vitamin B_2 (riboflavin) will also be accompanied by its more expensive and bioactive form: riboflavin 5-phosphate. Similarly, with vitamin B_6 (pyridoxine hydrochloride) a high-quality formula will also contain the more expensive and bioactive form: pyridoxol 5-phosphate.

No foolproof way exists to check out a vitamin product without knowing exactly what is going into the product: how old the ingredients are; how they have been shipped, handled and stored; and how pure they are. But taking those steps that you can do on your own will bring you closer to buying an effective product. (Vitamin products I have selected for my own use can be found in appendix C.)

Tasty Choices

The choices you face as you select a diet each day rests on a combination of the nutritional content of the foods balanced against your own personal tastes. Taste is acquired and is based largely on what we are familiar with. A new taste can be acquired simply by eating something new for a few weeks. I found that I lost my taste for a lot of the less desirable foods I used to enjoy. While taste and pleasure in eating are important (and even psychologically beneficial), plenty of healthy foods are pleasurable to eat.

Our productive, fast-paced, modern lifestyles, combined with misinformation about nutrition, can make the right choices difficult to identify. These lifestyles create a demand for processed, prepared, speedy "convenience foods," regardless of economic status or educational level. More parents than ever are working to support their families, while fewer and fewer are staying at home to tend gardens or prepare wholesome meals. Many of us no longer even eat at home. We eat in cafeterias, restaurants and fast-food chains where processed foods are the norm.

The food we ate yesterday is still affecting us today, and the food we eat at our next meal will affect our awareness, energy level, ability to think, learn and remember as well as our mood and behavior. What we eat in a week or a month or a year determines our biological makeup and our health, as well as the health of our children and grandchildren.

You must always remember that the biological reason for eating is to supply your cells with the nutrients they need on a daily basis. Becoming healthy and staying well with a diet of processed foods laced with sugar and processed oils is impossible. You are what you eat; your life and health depend on the foods you choose. You face these choices at every meal you eat for the rest of your life, so embrace it! You now know how to choose the good from the bad. Avoid the Big Four, eat "real" living food as nature provides and take high-quality supplements. To move yourself in the right direction on the nutritional pathway, start now to give your cells all the nutrients they need, every day, and they will thank you with the gift of good health.

6

THE TOXIN PATHWAY

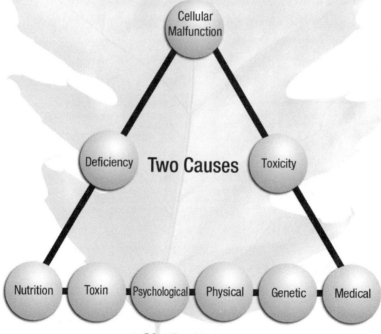

One Disease

Cellular Malfunction

Deficiency **Two Causes** Toxicity

Nutrition Toxin Psychological Physical Genetic Medical

Six Pathways

READER/CUSTOMER CARE SURVEY

We care about your opinions! Please take a moment to fill out our online Reader Survey at **http://survey.hcibooks.com**.
As a **"THANK YOU"** you will receive a **VALUABLE INSTANT COUPON** towards future book purchases as well as a **SPECIAL GIFT** available
only online! Or, you may mail this card back to us and we will send you a copy of our exciting catalog with your valuable coupon inside.
(PLEASE PRINT IN ALL CAPS)

First Name _____ MI. _____ Last Name _____

Address _____ City _____

State _____ Zip _____ Email _____

1. Gender
❑ Female ❑ Male

2. Age
❑ 8 or younger
❑ 9-12 ❑ 13-16
❑ 17-20 ❑ 21-30
❑ 31+

3. Did you receive this book as a gift?
❑ Yes ❑ No

4. Annual Household Income
❑ under $25,000
❑ $25,000 - $34,999
❑ $35,000 - $49,999
❑ $50,000 - $74,999
❑ over $75,000

5. What are the ages of the children living in your house?
❑ 0 - 14 ❑ 15+

6. Marital Status
❑ Single
❑ Married
❑ Divorced
❑ Widowed

7. How did you find out about the book?
(please choose one)
❑ Recommendation
❑ Store Display
❑ Online
❑ Catalog/Mailing
❑ Interview/Review

8. Where do you usually buy books?
(please choose one)
❑ Bookstore
❑ Online
❑ Book Club/Mail Order
❑ Price Club (Sam's Club, Costco's, etc.)
❑ Retail Store (Target, Wal-Mart, etc.)

9. What subject do you enjoy reading about the most?
(please choose one)
❑ Parenting/Family
❑ Relationships
❑ Recovery/Addictions
❑ Health/Nutrition
❑ Christianity
❑ Spirituality/Inspiration
❑ Business Self-help
❑ Women's Issues
❑ Sports

10. What attracts you most to a book?
(please choose one)
❑ Title
❑ Cover Design
❑ Author
❑ Content

FOLD HERE

Comments

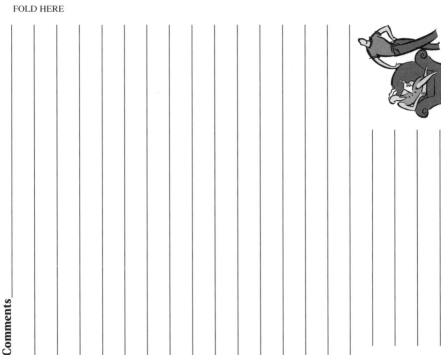

*"[O]ur health is threatened not only by individual chemicals
—deadly or toxic—but even more by the overall chemical load
that the human organism now has to sustain."*

Joseph D. Beasley, M.D., Ph.D.

The Kellogg Report

Our bodies are under attack every day—from without and from within. We face more toxic chemicals and man-made poisons in our lives than ever before. We are weakened by chronic stress, lack of exercise, allergies and eating the wrong foods in the wrong ways. In these ways, we often sabotage our own defense systems and invite the toxic enemy inside. If the enemy overpowers us, we fall—often without recognizing our attackers.

Toxicity—from toxins taken into our bodies from the outside or those created inside our bodies—is one of two reasons that cells malfunction; remember, toxicity is one of the two causes of disease. To prevent or to reverse disease, we must limit our exposure to toxins and we must give our bodies what they need to detoxify themselves. Fortunately, most of this process is within our control. Unfortunately, the invaders are everywhere—especially in our own homes—and often they are hard to find.

A Living Hell

By the time I received the telephone call from a man who identified himself as David, his body was losing its battle against an enemy he could not identify. "I have no idea who you are or why I am calling you," David said, "but I am going to kill myself."

My mind racing and my fear intensifying, I began the longest telephone conversation of my life—four and a half hours of David's life story, now a nightmare. Before the onset of his problems, David had been a partner in a top New York City advertising firm. He earned a seven-figure income and lived in a posh community; his wife was a socialite, and his children attended private schools. Life was good—until he began to experience weakness and fatigue. David went to see his physician, who did many thousands of dollars worth of testing, only to pronounce David to be in perfect health. The doctor's only suggestion was that David was working too hard and that he should take a vacation. So, David and his wife rented a house in Hawaii and stayed there for two months.

The vacation did not help, and David gradually felt worse. He developed serious allergies as well as neurological and psychological problems, so he consulted more doctors. A wealthy man, David went to the best doctors money could buy; they, too, could find nothing wrong, so they referred him to a psychiatrist. Physicians often assume that if they do not understand what is wrong, their ignorance is not at fault, but rather the patient is imagining the problem. David's psychiatrist was equally baffled, and he referred David back to his physicians.

All the while, David's fatigue and allergic symptoms worsened; he became unable to continue working and had to resign from his firm. Finally, David was referred to a clinical ecologist, a physician who specializes in environmentally caused diseases. This doctor diagnosed David as suffering from multiple allergies, chronic fatigue syndrome and chemical hypersensitivity syndrome. He said David was too chemically sensitive to continue living in the highly polluted New York area and suggested he move where air quality was better. David uprooted his family and moved to an isolated ranch outside of Santa Fe, New Mexico.

David's problems continued to worsen; he became dangerously depressed and irritable, and he had frequent outbursts of anger. David had descended into an unending nightmare, and he had taken his family with him. The combined impact of the move and the isolation, coupled with David's frequent outbursts of anger and his worsening depression, was too much for David's wife. She left him and she took the children with her.

Everything that David had ever cared about was gone. He was depressed, isolated and alone. He became suicidal. At that point, at the advice of a friend, he called me.

From the moment David called, I knew (in a general way) what his problem was. Diagnosing any disease is simple, because there is only one disease: malfunctioning cells. David's problem had to be a large number of malfunctioning cells, that much I knew. The critical questions were: Why were they malfunctioning, and how to restore them to normal function?

Four hours into our conversation, David provided a key piece of information that gave me the answer. David said he liked tuna fish, liked it so much that he typically ate two cans per day. This statement set off alarm bells in my mind because tuna fish contains a significant amount of mercury—a highly toxic heavy metal that poisons cells and deactivates key enzymes, causing numerous physical and mental problems, including suicidal tendencies.

Mercury pollution in our oceans bioaccumulates (gradually builds up) in fish and is especially concentrated in large fish such as tuna. In fact, the average can of tuna fish contains the maximum allowable daily dose of mercury, and David was eating two cans of tuna fish almost every day. Constant exposure like this results in a toxic bioaccumulation, so I began to suspect that mercury poisoning was at the root of David's problems.

His mercury exposure did not end with his taste for tuna; David had many silver amalgam dental fillings, and these amalgams contain about 50 percent mercury. His dental fillings (in addition to the tuna fish) had been exposing David to small amounts of mercury for most of his life. Finally, the straw that broke the camel's back was a dental procedure. David had to replace his aging mercury fillings and was exposed to high levels of mercury during this procedure because of the dentist's poor removal technique. This large exposure, combined with years of chronic, low-level exposure from the tuna fish and the dental fillings, was too much for David's body to handle. He fell into a state of toxic overload and his cells began to malfunction seriously.

David's failing health, chronic fatigue, emotional distress and suicidal tendencies were all symptoms of his toxic overload. The solution? I suggested nutritional supplements that would support David's natural ability to detoxify, and I also searched for and found a medical doctor who was an expert in mercury detoxification. Subsequently, David was cured of his mercury poisoning (through a process called chelation, which uses a chemical to react with the mercury and remove it from the body), and ultimately he was able to return to his life, his career and, most importantly, his family.

Killing Him Slowly

David is an excellent example of toxic overload in our modern society. He was chronically exposed to a specific toxin (mercury), which was slowly bioaccumulating in his cells. Already weakened by and sensitive to this toxin, he was suddenly exposed to a large amount, which pushed him over the brink. Another factor to be considered is David's bio-chemical individuality; he might have been born with a greater sensitivity to mercury than the average person. Virtually all Americans are now in a state of toxic overload. No wonder our population is becoming sicker and sicker. *Small toxic exposures each day (from common sources such as breakfast cereal, toothpaste, shampoo, soap, perfume, deodorant, hair dye, newspapers, magazines, exhaust fumes, carpets, new mattresses, dry cleaning or a newly painted bedroom) will increasingly exceed and even incapacitate your body's ability to detoxify, causing these chemicals to accumulate to a level that will make you sick.*

Man-made toxins are so prevalent today that they are impossible to avoid, regardless of where you live or what you do. Over the last one hundred years, we have introduced tens of thousands of man-made toxins to our environment, thus changing it dramatically. Our bodies are not genetically designed to deal with these levels and types of poisons that are accumulating in our tissues faster than we can rid ourselves of them.

Environmental toxins are not our only problem. We also generate powerful toxins inside our bodies. Unless we can minimize our exposure and maximize our bodies' detoxification systems, we will become sick. An extreme overload may even kill us:

- Only recently have researchers and health practitioners begun to understand the long-term effects of the thousands of chemicals we now encounter in our daily lives. At the time of my birth, the majority of these chemicals did not exist. Now they are all-pervasive.
- A growing body of scientific evidence links toxins to a wide variety of symptoms and syndromes, such as mental

and behavioral disorders, learning disabilities, fatigue, migraines, allergies, rashes and gastrointestinal disorders.

- Frightening new evidence suggests that low-level exposures to certain environmental chemicals are causing hormone disruptions, resulting in serious problems that range from birth defects to cancer.
- Many of the diseases that baffle our physicians (often called "diseases of aging" or "diseases of civilization") are the results of the toxic overload caused by modern industrialized society. These diseases are difficult to diagnose and impossible to cure using conventional medical approaches that just treat symptoms, rather than minimizing toxic exposure and optimizing detoxification.
- Chemicals posing little cancer risk can trigger cancer when combined together.
- Some chemicals and metals are toxic in any amount; others are beneficial or even essential in small amounts—such as vitamin A—but toxic in large amounts.

In the nineteenth century, less than 1 percent of all deaths in the United States were caused by cancer, and even at the turn of the twentieth century, only 3 percent of the population was affected. *Today, more than four in ten people will develop cancer in their lifetime, and one in four will die from cancer.*

The good news? Many of the strongest cancer-causing chemicals have been identified, and we can avoid them. The National Academy of Sciences sums up the challenge: "It is abundantly clear that the incidence of all the common cancers in humans is being determined by . . . potentially controllable external factors."

The Poisons Within

Toxins from the outside world—in our food, water, air, homes and workplaces—are known as *environmental toxins.*

Our bodies also manufacture a sea of internal toxins as a result of normal metabolism, which our bodies must eliminate in order to stay healthy. Few people realize that their own bodies can be a source of dangerous toxins—mostly in the digestive system, but also from allergic reactions, stress and other sources. Internal toxins are being generated at unprecedented rates as a result of modern diets, lifestyles and medical treatments. Just like an automobile produces exhaust, your body produces these toxins naturally and is designed to handle them; however, if abnormal amounts of toxins are produced or your ability to deal with them is impaired, you become sick.

Understanding the body's natural abilities to cleanse itself and how these abilities can be supported by diet, exercise and other means is important. By learning how to support your detoxification systems, you can reverse the effects of toxic overload; as toxic load decreases, cell function improves and disease often disappears.

Not all toxins, however, affect all people in the same manner. Just as each of us has unique needs for nutrients, each of us also has unique tolerances and susceptibilities to toxins. Toxin levels that can put one person into overload might not be particularly serious or even noticeable for someone else. Genetic predisposition, nutritional status, stress levels and lifestyle all influence toxin levels. Because currently we have no way to predict the effects that specific toxins (or combinations) have on any individual, the solution is to minimize exposure to all toxins and to take steps to support the body's detoxification mechanisms.

A Buildup of External Toxins

Chronic exposure to small amounts of seemingly harmless toxins presents a problem more dangerous than people realize. Even in trace amounts, toxins can build up and overload our cells, causing malfunction. The average American is building up (bioaccumulating) between three and five hundred man-made chemicals, most of which did not exist prior to World War II and have never before been in human tissue. Therefore, the combined toxic effects of these chemicals are impossible to calculate.

Physicians rarely consider toxic buildup as a primary cause of disease and rarely test for toxic underlying problems. In fact, about the only time the medical community will cite toxicity as a primary cause of disease is when somebody dies or becomes obviously ill from massive toxic exposure, such as a chemical spill. Subtle and gradual toxic exposures typically go undetected, which explains how people suffering from toxic overload can go to their doctors repeatedly (with persistent, if vague, complaints of "not feeling quite right") and never receive a correct diagnosis.

When people finally do become sick from their bioaccumulated toxins, following the path of their illness back to the myriad toxic sources is nearly impossible. If these toxins weren't so insidious and if they made us sick or killed us quicker and more straightforwardly, we would understand more readily the need to avoid them. Instead, we expose ourselves unknowingly and we lay the groundwork for massive cellular malfunction, little by little. Combine these external toxins with those generated inside the body, and the eventual result is toxic overload.

A chilling example: Environmental and dietary toxins bioaccumulate in a mother's fatty tissues throughout her life. When she starts nursing, her toxin-loaded fatty tissues produce cancer-causing breast milk. In his 1987 book *Diet for a New America,* John Robbins notes that the milk of most American mothers is so contaminated with chemicals (PCBs, dioxins and various pesticides) that "it would be subject to confiscation and destruction by the FDA were it to be sold across state lines." Robbins also says "the EPA has concluded that the average American breast-fed infant ingests nine times the permissible level of dieldrin, one of the most potent of all cancer-causing agents known to modern science." Fortunately, dieldrin, which was used on crops, has now been removed from the market, but the average mother's milk (while still far better than infant formula) remains contaminated with numerous toxic chemicals.

No One Is Safe

At present, toxic chemicals can be found in trace amounts in the tissues of virtually everyone in America—including you. These chemicals include: plastics such as styrene (disposable Styrofoam cups), 1,4-dichlorobenzene (mothballs, deodorizers), sodium lauryl sulfate (synthetic detergent from soaps, shampoos, toothpastes), pesticides, PCBs, dioxins, phthalates (plastics), formaldehyde (plywood, particleboard, permanent-press clothing), prescription drugs and organic solvents. No place on earth—and no modern home—is free from man-made toxic contamination. Molecules of the pesticide DDT, for example, blanket the entire planet.

Henry Schroeder, M.D., a former professor of medicine at Dartmouth Medical School and author of *The Poisons Around Us,* wrote that "five toxic trace metals: antimony, beryllium, cadmium, lead, and mercury are involved in at least half the deaths in the U.S. and much of the disabling disease." In all, more than one hundred thousand chemicals are now in commercial use, at least 25 percent of which are known to be hazardous; many others have never been tested at all!

Even when chemicals are tested for safety, studies are virtually always short-term and tested individually; few have examined the long-term effects of chemicals, or how they react in the body in combination with each other. Yet these long-term, combined effects are the reality of living in America today. In other words, the testing programs are flawed. Adverse effects are not necessarily observed in small groups of animals, nor do experimental animals necessarily react to toxins the same as humans. Ultimately, any chemical that is not normal and natural to our bodies puts a load on our detoxification systems and may damage cell function.

Most people make little effort to avoid toxins because officially established tolerances presume that toxin levels are within safe limits. Unless you make special choices, you constantly eat foods with trace toxins, you constantly drink water with trace toxins, you constantly use personal products with trace toxins, and you constantly breathe toxic air. By the end of each day, these toxic contaminants often reach a substantial cumulative total. EPA scientists found that *the total toxic residues in our daily diet can exceed 500 percent of the recommended daily maximum, even if each individual food is within "safe" limits!*

A Poison Gas Chamber of Her Very Own

Several years ago, a young married couple from Chicago asked me to help their three-year-old daughter, Anne, who was experiencing seizures. Anne had been examined by at least a dozen specialists, but their only recommendations were anti-seizure medications that made Anne sick, yet failed to stop the seizures. The desperate parents called me, a complete stranger two thousand miles away. They begged me for help, even though I am not a physician.

Because there is only one disease, I knew that Anne's problem was malfunctioning cells. But why were they malfunctioning? Although I asked many questions about Anne's history, nothing seemed unusual about her birth, background or development. She had been breast-fed (a good thing; even though breast milk is toxic, it is still preferable to the alternatives), and her diet was actually better than average. In fact, she had been remarkably healthy ever since birth—until the seizures started.

I began to ask questions about her environment. As it turned out, during most of her young life, Anne had been sleeping in a crib in her parents' bedroom. When she outgrew the crib, her parents decided she should have her own bedroom, and they refurbished a room. Knowing that brand-new room furnishings can be quite toxic, I focused on environmental toxins as the probable cause of the little girl's problems. I learned that before the onset of the seizures, Anne's new bedroom had been given a fresh coat of paint and was furnished with new wall-to-wall carpeting, a new television set and new furniture, including a new bed and mattress. In fact, that new bedroom had just about every amenity that any set of loving parents could give to their beloved daughter, but it was also a poison gas chamber! The new paint, carpet, mattress, television and furniture (constructed of particleboard, which contains formaldehyde) were all giving off toxic gases. You recognize the typical "new paint smell," that "new carpet smell" and that "new furniture smell." They are all toxic, especially when they are brand-new, at which time they emit higher concentrations of chemicals. Shut anybody inside a bedroom like little Anne's for eight or ten hours a night, and the person is exposed to a lot of toxins.

Anne was in toxic overload, and her seizures were the result. Often, in a case like this, when you remove the source of the toxins, you cure the disease. Instead, Anne's physicians had prescribed antiseizure medications, which added to her toxic overload, making her sicker. I suggested an experiment to Anne's parents: Close off the toxic bedroom and allow Anne to sleep in another room for a few weeks. The result: The seizures stopped, and Anne returned to being a normal and healthy child.

Fight Back with Foods

Why isn't our society taking more action to protect us from toxins? Why don't our physicians routinely warn us about toxins and check for them? One explanation lies in a 1988 report issued by the National Academy of Sciences titled, *Role of the Primary Care Physician in Occupational Environmental Medicine,* which concluded that while toxic environmental chemicals play an increasingly important role in modern chronic diseases, almost all physicians are ignorant about the degree to which low-level toxins affect health.

One of the most direct sources of our toxic exposures is the foods we eat. A meal that looks, smells and tastes good is a wonderful thing, but you owe your body more. You need to make sure your food is free of toxins and filled with nutrients that support your body's natural ability to detoxify. *You need to find out what is in your food, where your food came from and how your food has been altered from the way nature provided.*

One of the best ways to minimize the toxins is to buy organic foods. Organic is a method of growing and producing food free from chemical fertilizers and pesticides, artificial ripening agents, preservatives, genetic modification and radiation. The term "organic" applies to more than fruits, vegetables and grains; organically grown animals are fed organic feed and are produced without the customary use of antibiotics, hormones or other supplemental medications. Organic foods may be more expensive and somewhat more difficult to obtain, but they almost always contain fewer toxins and better nutrition. Read labels; the U.S. Department of Agriculture has approved organic certification and the label should bear the logo. Unless a product clearly says that it is organic, it almost certainly is not. If you live in an urban area, organic foods purchased at local farmers' markets are most likely the freshest, most nutritious, least toxic foods you can obtain. Despite that, almost 90 percent of the food dollars spent in America today are spent on toxic, processed foods that are not organic. To make matters worse, we eat almost no fresh food, limiting the nutrients available to help us detoxify all the bad stuff we constantly take in.

Feeding into Behavior Problems

Several years ago, a grandmother came up to me at a break in one of my workshops and asked what to do about her psychotic four-year-old grandson, Gerald. She described the boy's fits of uncontrollable anger and said that he would strike out at everyone and everything in his path. Gerald had been taken to a number of medical centers and examined by numerous physicians, who only offered powerful tranquilizers to calm the psychotic behavior. As is often the case, the prescribed drugs did not solve the problem; they just compounded it. The drugs made Gerald sick and lethargic, but did not eliminate his terrifying behavior.

The boy faced an uncertain future. That Gerald could ever be able to attend a regular school or hold a regular job seemed unlikely. I asked Gerald's grandmother many questions but was unable to find any obvious explanation for his psychotic behavior. One thing I learned about Gerald was that he drank a lot of milk and apple juice. Walking back to the podium to continue my presentation, I told the grandmother that while I honestly did not know what was wrong with her grandson, I did know that both milk and apple juice contain a lot of toxic chemical residues. Regardless of what was wrong, feeding him toxins was certainly not going to help him improve. I recommended a simple experiment: Stop feeding Gerald milk and apple juice.

About six months later, I was speaking at a meeting and, out of the corner of my eye, I spied Gerald's grandmother running toward me with an enthusiasm and a rate of speed that was almost alarming. She breathlessly exclaimed great news about the health of her grandson. Milk and apple juice were completely eliminated from the boy's diet, and he made a miraculous recovery. The psychotic behavior disappeared, and Gerald has been well ever since.

How the removal of milk and apple juice (two presumably

healthful foods) from a boy's diet could make such a difference is hard to imagine. We have no way, however, to know exactly how much damage the toxins in our food are causing. Too many factors are involved, and each person's biochemistry is unique. Some people, like this little boy, can be more sensitive to certain toxins, such as the ad exec David may have been to mercury. The solution, regardless of individual biochemistry, is to choose a diet that is low in toxins. A diet should consist of organic, fresh, whole/raw/unprocessed foods, pure water and avoidance of heavily processed/cooked foods.

Clean Up an Unrecognized Toxic Site: Your Pantry

The hard part is to obtain accurate information about what is good for you and what is not. A woman who had studied extensively in the fields of health and nutrition reminded me of this fact in a startling way. Even with her background, she had little understanding of how to select a nontoxic diet.

I met Cynthia at one of my all-day seminars. By the end of the day she was motivated to make major changes in her life and asked if she could purchase a day of my time so that I could teach her how to shop for healthful foods. Despite all of her previous study, she felt overwhelmed with information and confused about how to make healthy choices.

My day with Cynthia and her husband, Tom, serves as a general guide for you to start on a path toward a life-sustaining, nontoxic diet. The first thing I did with the couple was to clean out all toxic foods from their refrigerator and pantry. We ended up with several boxes filled with foods to be discarded; a lot of it was toxin-loaded breakfast cereal that her children would have eaten.

Then we headed to the local health food store. We went down each aisle and examined foods, read labels and discussed how to select foods that are either nontoxic or at least less toxic than supermarket alternatives. For example, a healthy substitute for the boxed cereals was found in the grain section of the health food store. We purchased a variety of organic, whole grains that could be cooked like rice and fed to the children. (By the way, the kids loved it.)

As Cynthia, Tom and I walked through the store, I began to explain principles that would help them in the future. Almost any type of food that has been packaged—in a box, jar, can or bottle—has been processed and is likely to contain toxic chemicals. These toxic chemicals either can be deliberately added to the foods (food additives), or they can result from food production practices (chemical residues). Whatever the source of these chemicals, processed foods (such as breakfast cereal, bread, canned foods, frozen foods, oils and vegetable shortenings, soft drinks, ice cream, cookies, cake and candy) are loaded with them. In addition to their lack of nutrition, the high toxic content in processed foods makes them a poor choice.

A variety of food additives are used to enhance flavor, color and texture; to help foods process better; and to extend their shelf life. In all, more than three thousand FDA-approved additives are in use today, and the average American ingests more than ten pounds of them per year. Imagining someone eating ten pounds of toxic, synthetic chemicals a year is diffi-cult, but we do it—a little at a time, without realizing how it adds up. Although food additives must be approved for safety, frequently they are initially determined to be safe, only to be removed later from the market due to unanticipated harmful effects. Do not assume that food additives are safe just because the FDA has approved them.

Furthermore, researchers usually test one additive at a time, even though we eat them in combination. Almost no research goes into studying the safety of food additive combinations. Our modern exposure to many different combinations of food additives is a gigantic and dangerous chemistry experiment. The combined toxic effects of food additives were reported in a study conducted by B. H. Ershoff (published in a 1976 *Journal of Food Science*) that examined three different FDA-approved food additives: an artificial color, an artificial sweetener and an emulsifier (a substance that keeps oil and water from separating). When fed one at a time, these food additives caused no readily observable side effects in experimental animals. But, when two of the additives were consumed at the same time, the animals became sick. When all three were combined, the test animals died in less than two weeks! Bearing this in mind, pick up an average box of breakfast cereal (or just about any other highly processed food) and count how many additives are in the product. Obviously, you are eating these additives in combination. After examining the labels on boxes of breakfast cereal in Cynthia and Tom's pantry, we discarded all of them because the labels showed that they contained artificial colors, flavors, preservatives and hydrogenated oils. *Read the labels on the foods that you buy. When a food contains artificial colors, flavors, preservatives or other additives, do not buy it.*

What would happen if we eliminated certain food additives from our diet? A study reported in a 1986 issue of the *International Journal of Biosocial Research* addressed this question. Between 1979 and 1983, the New York City public school system gradually removed foods containing artificial colors and flavors from the school lunches served to more than one million children. During this same period, without any other changes being introduced, the schoolchildren's academic performance skyrocketed. New York City schools experienced the largest four-year gain in academic performance ever measured in any city school district in U.S. history. How was such improvement possible? Food additives are toxic; they poison cells. When you stop poisoning cells, health improves. As the health of brain cells improves, so does the ability to think, learn and remember. A contributing factor to today's poor academic performance is the burden of toxic exposure on the developing minds of our young people. Unfortunately, once the experiment was over, because of political pressure from conventional food suppliers, the New York City schools reverted to "normal" foods, and these extraordinary gains were lost.

Another risk in processed foods you do not find on the label: toxic chemical residues. The manufacturer does not deliberately add these chemicals, but they are present in almost all ordinary commercial foods. If manufacturers do not add it, they do not have to list it. (Recall David's exposure to mercury in tuna fish; obviously, mercury is not listed on the label but it is in there, because it was in the fish.) Chemical residues come from many different sources, including industrial chemical and pesticide residues, herbicides, fungicides, artificial ripening agents, hormones and other veterinary drugs and packaging materials.

On our "tour" of hidden toxic residues, Cynthia, Tom and I took a walk down the frozen foods aisle. According to the 1982–1986 *FDA Total Diet Study,* frozen french fries contained 70 different pesticide residues. Frozen pizzas had 67 industrial and pesticide residues. Frozen chocolate cake contained 61 toxic residues and milk chocolate had 93. Peanut butter had a whopping 183, including highly carcinogenic aflatoxin, which is produced by a mold that grows on peanuts.

Lurking in all the aisles was another overlooked danger: packaging materials. The toxins in packaging materials (such as plastic wrap, plastic bottles, milk containers, juice boxes, Styrofoam and epoxy can linings) can leach toxins into our foods before we eat them. Foods coming into contact with packaging materials that contain water or oil-soluble toxic chemicals can absorb these chemicals, and then the consumer ingests them. Portions of the polymers, plasticizers, stabilizers, fillers and even colorants in plastic wrap can dissolve into the food. Avoid foods packaged in plastic. Choose foods packaged in more appropriate materials, such as paper and glass.

It's ironic that people sometimes spend extra money to buy organic foods, yet the foods may be wrapped in toxic packaging. Why purchase organic meat in a Styrofoam tray topped with plastic shrink-wrap, or organic canned goods in an epoxy-lined can? Unfortunately, these conveniences come at a price, and that price is the bioaccumulation of toxic chemicals in your body and subsequent disease.

Choosing Your Oils: A Slippery Slope

We continued our shopping trip, learning how to avoid foods that invite sickness. In the oils and salad dressings section, I reminded Cynthia and Tom that almost all oils on supermarket shelves are processed and toxic. These toxic oils also find their way into a variety of prepared and processed foods, including salad dressings, canned and baked goods.

Most oils, especially peanut, cottonseed and soybean, are highly contaminated with pesticide residues toxic to the nervous system. Many modern oils use chemical extraction methods, which leave solvent residues that are lung irritants, nerve depressants and detrimental to health in general. Even oils that have been cold-pressed (rather than chemically extracted) often are refined with toxic chemicals and exposed to high temperatures in their bleaching and deodorizing processes, making the oils toxic. Exposed to high temperatures, nutrients in these oils are altered and turned into toxic, trans-fatty acids and a variety of other toxins (aldehydes, ketones and hydroperoxides). About one-third of all the oil sold—whether bottled or contained in margarine, vegetable shortenings, baked goods, breakfast cereals, peanut butter, etc.—has been hydrogenated or partially hydrogenated and contains toxic trans-fatty acids and numerous other toxic chemicals.

Since these processed oils have come into widespread use, the incidence of myocardial infarction (a type of heart attack) has increased eightyfold, and heart disease, formerly rare, has become a leading cause of death. Coincidence? According to

Udo Erasmus, author of *Fats That Heal, Fats That Kill,* the
reason for these burgeoning health problems is that processed
oils promote a condition known as "fatty degeneration." In
this book, Erasmus wrote: "Sixty-eight percent of people die
from just three conditions that involve fatty degeneration: cardiovascular disease, cancer and diabetes." Only a handful of
healthful fats and oils are on the market: organic butter or
ghee, high-quality olive oil (difficult to find), and high-quality
essential fatty acid products such as flaxseed oil (see appendix
C for my personal choices).

Dangers in Dairy and Meat

Our little group arrived at the dairy section. As you recall,
milk and dairy products are not appropriate for human consumption and should be avoided by everyone, especially
infants and young children. Toxic bioaccumulation is a problem; virtually all of the toxins to which a cow is exposed during its life bioaccumulate in its tissues, and these toxins are
then present in its milk. You should regard milk as a toxic soup
filled with pesticides, antibiotics, dioxins, hormones, sulfa
drugs, tranquilizers and other contaminants. Worse, the practice of pasteurization (a heat treatment done to virtually all
milk products to kill bacteria) alters the physical and chemical
properties of the milk. Pasteurization not only renders the
nutrients less useful to your body but creates toxins as well.
Between the toxic bioaccumulation, the pasteurization and the
fact that milk products make up 25 to 50 percent of many
Americans' diets, milk is a major contributing factor to our
high rates of infectious, allergic and chronic disease. In fact,
milk consumption has been linked to many diseases, including
osteoporosis, multiple sclerosis, diabetes, heart disease and
cancer. My recommendation to Cynthia and Tom was that
they eliminate milk and milk products from their family
diet; I recommend the same to you. Milk does not do your
body good.

Animal products were our next stop. Meat and eggs can have serious toxicity problems. Though animal products contain essential nutrients (and I do not recommend a diet devoid of them), you must choose your sources carefully. The nutritional value of a food source should always be weighed against the toxins it contains or is likely to contain.

Commercial livestock contain many toxins, which become concentrated in their tissues. Foods from commercial cattle (and their milk), chickens (and their eggs) and most farmed fish are all poor food choices. All their lives, these animals are fed foods that are lacking in nutrition and toxic (contaminated with pesticides and other agricultural chemicals). Pound for pound, livestock feed is substantially more toxic than the foods we eat, not to mention that large animals like cattle eat a lot more food than we do. When you eat these highly toxic animals, or products derived from them, the toxins enter you. In 1976, the EPA studied human breast milk and found that the toxic contaminants in the milk of vegetarian mothers was only 1 to 2 percent of the national average. The solution is to minimize toxic exposure by selecting organically produced meat, poultry, eggs and wild fish from relatively nonpolluted deep-water ocean areas rather than those harvested from polluted coastal areas or farmed.

Selecting organically produced animal products almost certainly requires a trip to a well-stocked, reputable health food store. The foods are more expensive, but the extra money buys protection from toxins, as well as contributes to better nutrition and a more environmentally responsible method of farming.

Health is a choice. You can pay now for good food, or pay later for doctors and hospitals. If you cannot find ideal foods, however, often you can make better choices; if you cannot find high-quality (organic) animal products, then minimize your consumption. Remember that the overwhelming majority of our toxic pesticide exposure is from nonorganic animal products such as poultry, meat, eggs and milk products.

I do not recommend a totally vegetarian or vegan diet, because both lack essential nutrients; however, a primarily vegetarian diet is desirable. An organic vegetarian diet is the simplest and easiest way to minimize toxins and maximize your nutrient intake. When you eat animal products, select free-ranging, organic animal products whenever possible.

Anticipating Food Invaders

Toward the end of our shopping trip, I shared a fundamental yet largely unrecognized food shopping concept. *Selecting nontoxic foods means selecting foods that are not contaminated with bacteria and molds,* which produce toxins. When bacteria and molds contaminate our foods, they damage our health. As part of their normal metabolism, bacteria produce toxins that place a burden on the immune system and contribute to toxic overload, disease and even death. The most serious cases of bacterial food poisoning can result in death, such as the toxins produced by the *Clostridium botulinum,* the botulism bacteria (found mainly in improperly canned foods), the *E. coli* bacterium (found in improperly handled meat and a variety of other foods) and others, including the most common contaminations from staphylococcal and salmonella. Death from these infective pathogens is rare, but quite common is the exposure to low levels of bacterial toxins present in foods, particularly animal products. Always smell meat, fish and poultry. A rank, fishy or rotten scent means that the product is too old or has not been properly stored; bacteria are growing and producing toxins, and the oils are rancid and toxic. Never eat such foods.

Commercial milk products are contaminated with bacteria. Government regulations state that after pasteurization milk should contain no more than 20,000 bacteria per milliliter. Out of twenty-five milk samples analyzed by *Consumer Reports,* seven samples had in excess of 130,000 bacteria per milliliter;

one sample had almost 3,000,000; and other samples had too many bacteria to count! When you consider the toxins produced by these bacteria, combined with the toxins already present from agricultural and industrial sources, why would anyone still believe cow milk is good for infants and children?

Cynthia and Tom were familiar with the problems of bacterial contamination, but they, like most people, had almost no knowledge of the problems with mold. Not that mold problems are new: Stories from the Middle Ages tell of whole villages racing around in hallucinogenic madness after being poisoned by a type of mold, ergot, that grows on rye. Ergot produces a neurotoxin that poisons the brain and central nervous system. These sick people would sometimes go to a local monastery where the monks would take them in and pray for them—and they would be cured! How? The monasteries were built on better land at the tops of hills, whereas the farmers lived in the lowlands. When the monks harvested their grain on the hills, it was drier than the farmers' grain in the wet lowlands, hence less moldy. When the sick farmers ate uncontaminated grains, they became well. The bizarre behavior of children in Salem, thought to be witchcraft, now is thought to have been cause by ergotism. Although we do not run around in hallucinogenic madness today, at least not from food mold, the problem of mold in the food supply persists.

Molds can develop if crops are moist when harvested or stored. Food often spends weeks in the distribution process and becomes moldy by the time it reaches the store, even if it was not contaminated when harvested. Food has further opportunity to mold in your kitchen. Fresh, living plants protect themselves from mold growth (just as we humans have an immune system to protect ourselves from disease), but as food ages and dies, molds grow. People eat these moldy foods (especially when the mold is not visible), unaware of the toxic loads they put on their bodies. Worse, many people have become allergic to molds, causing not only a toxic exposure but also a toxic allergic reaction. In fact, people allergic to molds are often fine when they eat a freshly harvested berry or grape but suffer an allergic reaction when eating the same foods purchased in a grocery store. If you believe that a food is moldy, do not smell it. Inhaled mold causes serious health problems. Wrap the suspect food and dispose of it carefully.

Mycotoxins (toxins produced by molds) can injure and kill cells, and they are known causes of cancer, especially liver cancer. Because knowing the level of mold contamination in a particular food is difficult, the best approach is to avoid or minimize consumption of foods prone to becoming moldy, such as corn, nuts, grapes, raisins and all dried fruits, berries, beer and other fermented foods, and cheeses. Bottled apple juice frequently is moldy. Apple juice drinkers are so accustomed to its taste that they fail to recognize the presence of this toxin.

If you bite into a nut and it tastes bad, spit it out. It is toxic. If there is any visible mold on any part of a food, throw the entire food away. Don't just cut off the mold. When a mold infection takes place, foods naturally protect themselves by producing antimold toxins that are also toxic to you. Antimold toxins are produced throughout the food, not just the part you cut off. In general, susceptible products such as fresh berries must be purchased in season, freshly harvested from local growers; otherwise they are too old and too moldy—even if you cannot see the mold. I observe people in my local health food store purchasing a basket of "fresh" berries that already have visible mold. Obviously, they have no idea of how poisonous that is.

One type of mold that grows on grains and nuts (particularly corn, peanuts, walnuts and pistachios) produces a mycotoxin called aflatoxin, which is known to cause cancer. Although our government tries to regulate aflatoxin levels, highly contaminated crops are constantly finding their way into our food supply. The chilling reality is that aflatoxin is most commonly found in some of the foods that we most frequently feed to our children—corn flakes, other corn products, peanuts and peanut butter.

Some Cooking Methods Can Create Toxins

Once we obtain high-quality foods, we still must prepare them properly. The first step in nontoxic food preparation is to wash or peel foods in order to remove agricultural chemicals, bacteria and molds. Waxed foods (such as most cucumbers, eggplant, turnips and apples) definitely should be peeled, because the wax often is covering surface residues of pesticides and fungicides that are applied before the wax is applied; also, questions abound about the safety of some of the waxes. For foods that cannot be peeled, washing under running water for a minute or two does a relatively good cleaning job; using a pure, liquid castile soap (a mild soap made from olive oil and sodium hydroxide) cleans even better. For foods like lettuce, discard the outer layers and wash the leaves separately. Rinsing briefly in a vinegar solution lowers bacteria levels.

Few people are going to eat 100 percent of their diet raw (I eat about 80 percent of mine raw), but whenever you choose to eat a raw food in place of a highly cooked or processed one, you obtain better nutrition and less toxic exposure. Cook foods lightly. Ideally, food should not be cooked at temperatures higher than boiling water or steam. Foods change fundamentally when they are cooked; they can become more toxic, less nutritious and even more difficult to digest. *Avoid browned or charred foods, which are highly toxic.* Unfortunately, many Americans have developed a taste for charbroiled, toasted or barbecued foods, which develop mutagens that contribute to cancer.

When food is heated above 375 degrees (as it usually is in toasting, frying, grilling, broiling and barbecuing), a number of toxic compounds can be produced, including heterocyclic aromatic amines (HAAs). HAAs are among the most powerful carcinogens ever discovered, and even minute amounts of them can damage your DNA.

The rule of thumb is that the higher the temperature and the longer the cooking time, the more HAAs are formed. Thus, medium rare is safer than well done, and blackened foods are absolutely not acceptable. If ever I am served food that is black, I cut off the blackened parts. Even toast is dangerous. Experiments at Lawrence Livermore Laboratory showed that a well-toasted piece of bread had 20 percent of the cancer-causing activity of a well-done hamburger. Dosage and frequency are the problems; many people eat several slices of toasted bread or bagel every morning for breakfast, which is like laying out a welcome mat for cancer.

Microwaves: A Fast Track to Trouble

Cooking food is not a good idea, especially at high temperatures, but cooking in microwave ovens may be even worse. While not browning or blackening food like conventional cooking, microwaving changes the chemistry of food fundamentally, lowering nutritional content and producing unique toxins. A lot more goes on inside a microwave than just making things hot. Microwaves "zap" food with enormous amounts of energy—enough to break apart water molecules and cause them to react with the food in ways they would not do otherwise. These reactions create a lot of strange, new molecules that are unnatural to the human body; some of them are toxic and carcinogenic. Research in Switzerland, the former Soviet Union and the United States all suggest that eating microwaved food may promote certain types of cancers, hormone imbalances, lymphatic disorders, digestive disorders, immune and blood abnormalities, emotional problems, permanent brain damage, and even heart disease.

In 1992, at the Swiss Federal Institute of Technology, volunteers who ate microwaved food experienced decreased hemoglobin content of their blood and an increased white cell count. Thus, microwaved food decreases the amount of oxygen available to our cells and stresses the immune system. Also, microwaves have been demonstrated to damage nutrients. Research at the Institute of Radio Technology at Kinsk, in the former Soviet Union, found that microwaves reduce the nutritional content of food by 60 to 90 percent. When reheating food, use the stovetop or oven. Modern foods are already nutrient deficient. Why make them worse by using a microwave?

Use the right cookware. The best pots and pans are those made of glass or ceramics such as Corning Ware. Other materials interact with foods and introduce some level of toxins into the food. Stainless steel contains nickel—both an allergen and a carcinogen. A study in the *Journal of the American Dietetic Association* found that toxic chemicals from stainless steel pots, including nickel, iron and chromium, enter food during cooking. Aluminum—from pots, pans and aluminum foil—is another toxic contaminant. Teflon coatings on cookware also present problems, especially when such cookware is heated to higher temperatures.

Of course, not all meals come from your own kitchen. Americans eat an enormous percentage of food at restaurants. Making optimal food choices when eating at restaurants is almost impossible. However, with care in menu selection, you can usually do fairly well. As a rule of thumb, upscale restaurants usually have fresher and better prepared foods, while fast-food restaurant offerings are more toxic and less nutritious. Many restaurants do not even "cook" for you; they merely serve prepared and processed foods that are reheated (perhaps in a microwave, so be sure to ask).

Very few restaurants use high-quality organic meats. Bear this in mind the next time you ponder a menu. Deep-water ocean fish is probably your best choice, but only if it is fresh. Fresh-water fish is likely to be contaminated with toxins, and farmed fish are neither nutritious nor free of toxins. When ordering out, I often select large salads or freshly harvested· fish, with vegetables. Many restaurants are willing to make up a vegetarian entrée on request. Avoid anything that is "black-ened," as well as selections containing meat and, particularly, dairy products. Make simple selections, and be able to iden-tify all the ingredients.

Caution: This Water Is Hazardous to Your Health

In addition to food, water is an essential ingredient for life and good health. Adequate water intake helps rid your body of toxins, both through the kidneys and through sweat. Shockingly, however, in a highly developed nation such as the United States, almost all of the water is toxic; it adds poisons to your body and is unfit to drink.

Toxins from landfill runoff, sewage pollutants, industrial chemicals such as PCBs and vinyl chloride, agricultural runoff (particularly pesticides), leakage from gasoline storage tanks, and other pollutants contaminate our water. Some researchers believe chronic low-level exposure to these chemicals con-tributes to our cancer epidemic. Even those of us fortunate enough to live near a high-quality water source would prob-ably be disappointed to learn that our local water supplier takes perfectly good water and contaminates it with toxins such as chlorine, fluoride, arsenic and aluminum. Water then travels through municipal and household pipelines, which can add contaminants such as lead, cadmium, copper, asbestos, iron and nickel.

Although these toxins exist in minute amounts, we drink water (or beverages made with water) daily, so we are exposed chronically. This exposure leads to toxic bioaccumulation, cellular malfunction and disease. Minimize tap-water con-sumption; drink high-quality distilled or spring water (prefer-ably in glass containers to avoid toxins from plastics). Purchase from companies willing to provide you with a chemical analysis of their water. Another alternative is to drink tap water purified by a filter that uses reverse osmosis. Remember that commercial fruit juices and other beverage products are usually made with tap water. Pure water is what your body needs; when you can get it, choose it.

What Is in Your Drinking Water?

How do some of the toxins commonly added to municipal water supplies harm your health? About 80 percent of the drinking water in the United States is chlorinated. Chlorine is an extremely toxic and volatile chemical that reacts with organic matter in tap water to form carcinogenic compounds called trihalomethanes. These compounds bioaccumulate in fatty tissues and are capable of causing genetic mutations, suppressing immune function, and interfering with the natural controls of cell growth. Long-term consumers of chlorinated water have been shown to have higher risks of rectal, bladder, kidney, intestinal, liver, pancreatic and urinary tract cancers, as well as spontaneous abortions. The Department of Health Services in California reports that women who drink bottled or filtered water have substantially lower rates of birth defects and miscarriages compared to women who drink tap water. Just opening the tap to wash your hands releases toxic chlorine fumes that, when breathed, damage your health; taking a shower is many times worse. I use a charcoal filter in my shower to filter out the chlorine and organic pollutants.

Fluoride is more toxic than lead and only slightly less toxic than arsenic, yet we have been conditioned to believe that fluoride is good for us. Presumably, we put fluoride in our water to prevent tooth decay. Although tooth decay has indeed declined worldwide since the 1970s—an event for which fluoride is often wrongly credited—the real reason for the decline remains unknown, because tooth decay has declined at the same rate in countries that do not use fluoride. Most people are unaware that in more than fifty years of testing and widespread use, no one has ever been able to prove that fluoride is either safe or effective, which is why fluoride has never been approved by the FDA. After half a century of use, the FDA still classifies fluoride as an "unapproved new drug." Once again, we are guinea pigs in a vast medical experiment gone awry. The truth is, fluoridation of drinking water is making us sick, but no one is ready to admit it because of the almost unthinkable legal liability. Do you think it is a coincidence that toothpastes now have toxicity warnings about their fluoride content? Many young children swallow toothpaste, unless supervised by adults.

The truth about fluoride is gradually being revealed; a number of large-scale studies suggest that fluoride does not prevent and may even cause dental problems. Fluoride bioaccumulates in the body and has been shown to damage teeth, bones, kidneys, muscles, nerves, genes and immune function. In fact, fluoride toxicity is causing diseases such as dental and skeletal fluorosis. Dental fluorosis is a malformation of tooth enamel characterized by brittleness and discoloration, ultimately damaging the health of the teeth. Dentists tell people that fluorosis is "merely" a cosmetic problem. In reality, fluorosis is a sign of systemic fluoride poisoning. More than one out of five U.S. schoolchildren now have some degree of dental fluorosis, and X rays of children with dental fluorosis often show bone abnormalities (skeletal fluorosis) elsewhere in the body. Skeletal fluorosis weakens bones in a manner similar to osteoporosis. Early stages usually are misdiagnosed as arthritis, and advanced stages usually are misdiagnosed as osteoporosis. The minimum crippling fluoride dosage (the dosage that can cause skeletal fluorosis) is 5 milligrams per day for twenty to forty years, according to the National Academies for the Advancement of Science, yet Americans living in fluoridated areas average up to 6.6 milligrams per day!

Fluoride is a powerful enzyme poison that fundamentally

damages cell function, thereby causing disease and death. Mortality rates are higher in fluoridated communities. A 1978 study in the *New England Journal of Medicine* found that: "This pattern of a higher crude death rate in the cities with fluoridated water supplies was apparent for all categories of death except for those by accidental means and suicide." According to Dr. William Marcus, a senior scientist at the EPA, fluoride is the only substance known to cause bone cancer, and bone cancer rates are 80 to 600 percent higher in communities with fluoridated water. Similarly, new research connects fluoride intake to Alzheimer's disease by implicating a reaction that happens between aluminum and low-dose fluoride. Most home water filters do not remove this toxin. You need to use reverse osmosis or buy bottled water that does not contain fluoride.

Another toxin in our drinking water is arsenic. Arsenic, a contaminant in the chemicals used to fluoridate water, is known to cause cancer and to damage the digestive, cardiovascular, neurological, reproductive and immune systems. Aluminum salt (alum) is added to water to "purify" it by helping to settle and remove particulate and organic matter. A study in the *Journal of Epidemiology* found that the risk of developing Alzheimer's is increased in individuals who drink water with high aluminum concentrations.

Foods That Tamper with Destiny

No discussion of food toxins would be complete without mention of the potential for poisoning the entire population with genetically modified foods. Genetic engineering is the process of disrupting the genetic blueprints of living organisms by inserting genetic information from other organisms to obtain some "desirable characteristic," such as resistance to herbicides or insects. These foods are novel and totally unnatural, and we have no idea what the future health consequences may be, yet avoiding genetically modified foods is difficult.

Insertion of genes into genetic material is not a precise process. It is all too easy to obtain unintended results that lower nutritional content, create harmful allergens or lead to the creation of unique toxins. The effects of these toxins may not become known for years, while irreparable harm is being done. The best way to avoid these foods is to eat organically produced foods. (More on this subject in chapter 9, on the genetic pathway.)

Beware of the Air in Your Home

We have already discussed how toxic your food pantry and cupboards may be, but your home—while it may be your castle—may be more like a toxic waste dump. In fact, our greatest exposure to volatile organic compounds occurs in the home. Toxicity from indoor air pollution affects most Americans' health to some degree and produces a wide variety of symptoms, including anxiety, depression, fatigue, headaches, poor concentration and mental acuity, and bodily aches and pains. When people complain of these symptoms to their doctor, however, indoor pollutants are almost never suggested as a probable (or even possible) cause.

Learn to recognize toxins in your home. *Seemingly benign items can produce dangerous toxins that pollute your indoor air,* such as the off-gasses of mattresses, pillows, televisions, clothes, furniture, carpets and tap water. Toxins from these sources expose us to even higher concentrations than outdoor air pollution. In fact, the level of indoor pollutants in your home may be hundreds of times greater than outside air. Because most Americans spend about 90 percent of their time indoors, this toxic load can substantially contribute to toxic overload, resulting in disease.

As mentioned earlier, I used to suffer from an extreme case of multiple chemical sensitivities, and I was easily incapacitated by exposure to even minute quantities of toxins in my own home. I was able to restore my health only after years of minimizing toxins and improving my nutrition. One of the most profound things I learned from my illness is that all of us are chemically sensitive in varying degrees. This experience led me to research how the fumes from cleansing agents, air fresheners, fragrances and body care products injure our delicate detoxification mechanisms and use up the body's nutrient reserves that are required to operate these systems and prevent toxic damage.

There are multiple sources of indoor pollutants: new carpets, new paint, household cleansers, furniture, mattresses, copy machines, printers, electronic equipment, dry cleaning, newspapers and magazines. Anything you can smell that is not a natural smell is probably toxic. The longer you breathe it, and the more concentrated it is, the more damage it inflicts. Indoor air is a health risk because of the combined effects of multiple toxic sources concentrated in a confined space.

Few people know better the incredible amount of damage that can be done by indoor air pollution than Sally, a young newlywed. Sally was truly "brought" to my office. Her husband had to carry her from their car. She did not have enough energy to walk or even to hold her head up straight while seated. Sally was suffering from acute chronic fatigue, a condition that physicians are not trained to recognize or understand. She and her husband had already spent many thousands of dollars on consultations with physicians and diagnostic tests. Unable to find anything "physically wrong," Sally's doctors referred her to a psychiatrist.

Of course, Sally was not crazy, but she was very sick. Her cells were malfunctioning so badly that she had become totally disabled. The couple's responses to my questions, in addition to my own experience with chemical sensitivity, allowed me to understand what was wrong. First (like most of us), Sally had frequently been given antibiotics throughout her life. (Antibiotics cause fundamental and damaging changes to human physiology.) This intake resulted in a heightened susceptibility to environmental toxins. I asked many questions about Sally's medical history, diet, lifestyle and environment before focusing on the toxin pathway as the most important factor.

Sally was a writer, and her husband had converted their oversize laundry room into an office for her. Also in that room was a gas-fired water heater. Natural gas appliances release toxic gases, including nitrogen dioxide, carbon monoxide and small amounts of the natural gas itself. With insufficient ventilation, the gases became concentrated, and poor Sally was breathing them all day long. She began to suffer from sore throats, eye irritations, respiratory problems, headaches and, eventually, chronic fatigue.

I recommended they install an electric hot water heater. Sally's worst symptoms immediately were alleviated, although significant damage had already been done (both by the gases and the antibiotics). Her health was restored eventually after she worked to reverse the damage through improved diet and nutritional supplementation.

One of the great joys in my life is to watch someone like Sally go from being sick and disabled, with little to look forward to, to smiling once again and enjoying life. I am saddened to think how many people remain sick because their physicians do not understand the toxin pathway and have no idea how to help them. In fact, physicians who prescribe antibiotics and other medications often create susceptibility to such problems in the first place.

Gas-fired appliances (hot water heaters, ovens, stoves, furnaces, fireplaces or clothes dryers) diffuse toxic gases into the surrounding air. If you have such appliances, try to keep them out of your living space and put furnaces, clothes dryers and water heaters in a garage, shed or breezeway along with stored volatiles such as paints and cleaning fluids. A gas stove, because it is in your living space, should be replaced or at least very well ventilated. In my own recovery process, I had to convert from a gas to an electric water heater because I had become so sensitive to these toxins.

Giving off toxic gasses is an especially common problem with products when they are new. At one of my seminars, a woman named Diane raised her hand and explained that she was suffering from splitting headaches. After hearing the story about Sally, Diane realized that her headaches coincided with the purchase of a new car; she suspected a connection. Her new car was off-gassing toxins, producing the "new car" smell. Diane's family had two cars, so I suggested that she drive the older car until the odor subsided. Her headaches went away. Some highly sensitive people retrofit their cars with safer materials.

Consider the risk of new products: a new carpet, a freshly painted room, a new TV set, a new mattress. New products give off high levels of toxic chemicals. With the passage of time, the volume of toxic chemicals being off-gassed drops dramatically. Often you can accelerate the off-gassing process simply by applying heat. For example, the chemicals contained in a new car's plastics, adhesives and seating materials pollute the interior air of the car. During the first few months, try to leave a new car parked in the hot sun with the windows up to bake out the toxins. Air it out regularly, and be sure to air it out before and while you drive.

The risk of new paint is something my friend Jim discovered when he went from being generally in good spirits to suffering the worst depression of his life. Actually, he felt suicidal. I immediately tried to isolate the cause of Jim's malfunctioning cells. I discovered that Jim just had the interior of his house painted; paint off-gasses neurotoxins that can affect moods and mental function. New paint takes at least two months to reach reasonable levels of safety for most people (depending on biochemical individuality), which is why it is best to paint only one room at a time and to close freshly painted rooms off as much as possible while they are off-gassing. *Absolutely do not sleep in a freshly painted room!* A good idea is to schedule painting just before leaving on a vacation. Jim stayed at his son's house for several weeks, and his problem was solved.

Another example of toxic off-gassing was brought to my attention when a woman suffering flulike symptoms came to me for help. Ellen Marie had "caught the flu" around Christmas time the previous year and still was not well. Her physicians were dumbfounded, as anyone would be if they focused only on mitigating her symptoms.

I discovered that Ellen Marie had moved into a newly con-structed luxury home four months prior to coming down with "the flu." Her new home was constructed with particleboard, which off-gasses formaldehyde—a highly toxic and carcino-genic chemical. Plywood also will off-gas formaldehyde, but far less of it. (Some new man-made building materials no longer contain formaldehyde, but the substitutes used, such as iso-cyanates, are also toxic.) This poor woman was suffering from subtle and constant formaldehyde poisoning. Her symptoms included immune suppression, respiratory problems, coughing, throat irritation, headaches, insomnia, nausea and fatigue. I sug-gested to Ellen Marie that she sell her new home and move to a safer environment. She chose not to move and she remained ill. *Always select building materials and furniture that are made from real wood or at least plywood, but not particleboard.*

Inventory Your Home's Hazards

Do you have carpets in your home and, if so, from what are those carpets made? Carpets made from synthetic fibers (plastics such as nylon, acrylic or polyester), especially when new, off-gas large amounts of toxins. Carpets are among the most significant contributors to the toxicity of indoor air. The plastic fibers used to make carpets are very thin, thus creating an enormous amount of surface area from which off-gassing can occur. Chemicals used in the adhesive backing and those in the foam padding underlayer also off-gas. Carpets are treated with toxic soil and stain repellents, moisture repellents, mothproofing and other finishes. These chemicals are effective for their intended purposes, but toxic—an important consideration if you are looking for new floor coverings or considering a move into a newly carpeted space. *That "new carpet smell" is toxic, and the best solution is to use carpets made only of natural fibers* (wool is a good choice, though make sure it is not treated with toxic mothproofing chemicals). Hardwood or tile floors with natural-fiber area rugs are good alternatives.

How about the air quality in your bedroom, which you typically breathe for eight consecutive hours every day? What is the composition of your mattress? We spend one-third of our lives in bed, and spending most of that time immediately next to even mildly toxic chemicals can take a huge toll. Most mattresses today are made of synthetic materials (polyester, polyurethane, treated with dyes, flame retardants, etc.), which can off-gas for years and poison you while you are sleeping. Fortunately, 100 percent natural mattresses are available. Also, with a doctor's prescription you can obtain mattresses manufactured without toxic flame retardants that otherwise are required by law. At the very least, if you purchase a standard mattress, put it in the garage and allow it to off-gas for a few months before sleeping on it. Also, enclose the mattress with a thin polyethylene drop cloth or a tightly woven barrier-cloth that limits the amount of toxins you breathe nightly. Also, use pillows made from natural materials, such as down.

Next, look in your bathrooms. It's likely that enough toxic chemicals are there to make anybody sick. The toxic products include not only toilet bowl cleaners and air fresheners, but items such as toothpaste, mouthwash, hair spray, cosmetics, shampoo and soap (not to mention the toxic chlorinated water coming out of the tap). All of these products can be replaced with safer, simpler items available in health food stores; they will be equally effective without harming your health.

The laundry room is another toxic site. Detergents, bleach, spot removers and fabric softeners all contain chemicals that are toxic to you and to the environment. Manufacturers have lulled us into complacency with the term "biodegradable detergents." This fact has little to do with the eventual health and environmental impact of these synthetic chemicals. Biodegradable means only that at some point the detergent will lose its foaming properties. Purchase unscented products. Detergents can be replaced with soap-based products, while bleach can be replaced with safer sodium percarbonate or hydrogen peroxide.

Furniture anywhere in the house, but especially in bedrooms, can present significant risks. Today, furniture often is made with toxic synthetic materials (polyester, polyurethane, polystyrene and polyvinyl chloride), which off-gas toxic vapors; likewise, some types of furniture are made of particleboard (which, as already mentioned, will off-gas formaldehyde) and then covered with a wood or plastic veneer. Alarmingly, most children's furniture is made with toxic particleboard! One study showed that introducing particleboard furniture into an empty house tripled the formaldehyde levels in the air. This problem can be particularly acute in mobile homes, where *everything* may be made from particleboard. Buy furniture made from natural materials, such as solid wood or metal furniture; if this option is too expensive, consider used furniture made of these materials.

Even the clothes you wear can be toxic. Have you ever gone into a clothing store and noticed the chemical-laden atmosphere? Most clothes today contain or are made of toxic synthetic fibers (such as nylon, polyester, acrylics and spandex), which will affect you adversely as you wear them and also contribute to toxic indoor air. Clothes are often treated with dyes, formaldehyde finishes (permanent press), and mothproofing pesticides. Dry cleaning clothing brings toxins into your household and close to your body; clothes that have been dry-cleaned should always be aired out before they are put into a closet or worn. Laundry detergents and fabric softeners can also be problematic; in fact, many people are quite sensitive to detergent residues. Have you ever walked down the detergent aisle at the grocery store and had your eyes, nose or throat feel irritated? Toxins in those boxes are off-gassing. When washing your clothes, use environmentally friendly and unscented laundry products available in health food stores. Do not use scented fabric softeners. These products might make your clothes smell "fresh and clean," but that smell is toxic. *Buy clothes made of natural materials, such as wool and cotton, and use natural cleaning products.*

After you have taken steps to reduce or eliminate products that are toxic, *make sure to also* keep your home or office well ventilated. Modern homes and office buildings are built a lot "tighter" than older construction to save on energy costs. While reducing energy waste is a good thing, reducing air circulation allows pollutants to accumulate to higher concentrations. For this reason, high-quality air filters (that will filter out both particulate matter and gaseous hydrocarbons) can be helpful. Use them in rooms where you spend a great deal of time, such as your office or bedroom.

Obvious as it sounds, the most important thing you can do to keep your indoor air clean is to stop introducing pollutants in the first place. Before you purchase something new, consider if that product might contribute to your indoor pollution. As mentioned earlier, after you buy something, give it a chance to off-gas before you put it in your living environment. When I purchase a new television or computer monitor, I put it in the garage, turn it on and leave it there until I can no longer detect an odor. Hang your dry-cleaning outdoors or in a well-ventilated area until you can no longer detect an odor. Do not use products that have powerful chemical odors, such as mothballs or air fresheners. Use heat or sunshine to help expedite the off-gassing process, whenever possible.

Health and Beauty Products That Fail

Your skin provides enormous protection from microorganisms, such as germs, but skin also is designed to be permeable, allowing certain molecules in and out, which is good news when the skin allows antioxidants in to protect against the sun and allows toxins out through the sweat and oil glands. However, easy access also allows environmental toxins to penetrate.

Personal care products are the largest source of toxic absorption through the skin and mucus membranes. One study found that 13 percent of the commonly used cosmetic preservative BHT (butylated hydroxytoluene) is absorbed by your skin. Chemicals found in everyday personal products such as perfume, cologne, shaving cream, skin lotions, aftershave, toothpaste, soaps, shampoos, deodorants, nail polish, all types of household cleansers and so forth, can be absorbed quickly and produce effects that are toxic or even carcinogenic, especially when these toxic substances are combined.

When I was suffering from severe chemical sensitivities, I found, much to my surprise, that the brands of toothpaste, shampoo, deodorant and skin lotion that I was using were all quite toxic. Products such as lotions, conditioners and makeup, especially when left on the skin for long periods of time, expose you to significant amounts of toxins, which can bioaccumulate, poison your cells and cause disease. Most common products sold to preserve and protect the skin in fact actually contain chemicals capable of damaging the skin.

Virtually all commonly available cosmetic and personal care products contain ingredients (such as preservatives and colors) that are known to present problems. Many preservatives contain or release formaldehyde, a known toxin and carcinogen. Various parabens (a specific class of preservatives) have been shown to damage deep layers of the skin worse than severe sunburn, which causes the skin to age prematurely and even can cause cancer. Artificial colors have been shown to be carcinogenic, not only when ingested but also when applied to the skin. Yet people voluntarily put these personal care products on their skin daily, unaware that these products contain toxic and potentially carcinogenic ingredients. *By using products such as sunscreen and lotion, people are putting cancer-causing chemicals on their skin, then wondering why they developed skin cancer or why their skin is aging so fast.*

Choosing safe personal care and cosmetic products means reading labels carefully and learning about the health consequences of ingredients. Effective products are on the market that are high in quality and safety. The overwhelming majority, however, contain a variety of toxins that should be avoided. Some of the common toxins to look for and avoid include artificial fragrances, colors and flavors, formaldehyde, phenol, trichlorethylene, BHT/BHA, EDTA, cresol, detergents, glycols, parabens, sodium lauryl sulfate and nitrates/ nitrosamines.

Perfumes and other fragrances also cause problems. Traditionally, these products were made from flowers and herbs. But since World War II, most fragrances and perfumes have been made from synthetic petrochemicals, many of which are officially designated as hazardous materials. In fact, about 95 percent are synthetic, and more than 80 percent of the ingredients used in fragrances have never been tested for human safety. When they have been tested, many are found to be neurotoxic and even carcinogenic. (Meanwhile, because of "trade secrets," manufacturers are not required to list any of these toxic ingredients on their product labels.) Worse, these fragrances are not just in perfumes, but in everything from kitty litter to shampoos, soaps, lotions, shaving creams, household cleaners, laundry detergents and numerous other products. Fragrances now pollute our homes, schools, workplaces, stores, churches and other public places. People who regularly use synthetic perfumes are putting a heavy toxic burden on their bodies. The solution is to use essential oils made from natural ingredients such as flowers and herbs, if tolerable, and to avoid household and personal products made with synthetic fragrances.

I have spent years researching the toxic effects of chemicals used to make products that people consume on a daily basis. I discovered that regular toothpaste, for example, contains numerous toxins, such as fluoride, artificial colors, flavors, sweeteners and synthetic detergents, all of which can bioaccumulate in the body and lead to toxic overload. Toothpaste is especially important because the mucous membranes in your mouth are very permeable, so if you expose yourself to toxic toothpaste several times a day, you subject yourself to a lot of toxins. I eventually selected a toothpaste for my personal use that was both safe and effective (see appendix C), but it took eighteen months of research to find it.

Toxic chemicals, used for detergent and foam-generating properties, are present in most toothpastes, as well as in many other personal care and household products. When these toxins—sodium lauryl sulfate, sodium cetyl sulfate and sodium laureth sulfate—are placed on the surface of the body, they can cause eye irritations, skin rashes, hair loss, scalp flaking similar to dandruff and allergic reactions. These chemicals are known to be irritating to the skin and are used to irritate the skin in laboratory experiments! Think about what happens when your highly sensitive gum tissue comes into contact with a known irritant, like sodium lauryl sulfate, in your toothpaste. Could this factor be contributing to our epidemic of gum disease?

These man-made detergents pass through the skin and mucous membranes and bioaccumulate in fatty tissue—eye tissue, for example. Is there a possible connection between the sodium lauryl sulfate found in toothpaste and our epidemic of macular degeneration—a disease in which cells in the central part of the retina degenerate, and the leading cause of blindness in people over age fifty-five?

The focus of manufacturers is always on marketability, so they often try to disguise these synthetic and toxic ingredients by making them seem "natural." Labels will often state something like, "sodium lauryl sulfate—derived from coconut." Regardless of derivation they are toxic and can accumulate easily in your tissues to levels that cause cellular malfunction and disease.

People choose antibacterial soaps thinking they will protect them from germs, but the germicide in the soap goes right through the skin and bioaccumulates in tissue. In fact, these toxic chemicals, designed to kill cells, are now showing up in alarming amounts in human breast milk, and infants are much more susceptible to toxins. As always, the solution is to choose safe, natural products, usually available at health food and specialty stores. There are high-quality, certified organic, hair and skin care products available and I recommend you use them. (See appendix C for my personal choices.)

Toxic Cleaning Products

The home can be a toxic place already—do not make it more so with toxic cleaning products, solvents and workplace chemicals. Household cleaning products rank among the most toxic everyday substances to which people are exposed. Unfortunately, the manufacturer of household products is seldom the best source of accurate information about safety. As a practical matter, do not let any chemical come in contact with your skin unless you know it is safe. Most commercial brands are not safe, although safe household products are available at health food and specialty stores. (See appendix C for my choices.)

Some especially toxic household cleaners include ammonia,

chlorine bleach, aerosol propellants, detergents, petroleum distillates and toluene. Many of these substances not only harm the skin; they also give off toxic fumes that affect the person using the product and everyone else in the household. If you cannot avoid toxic household products, at least use them sparingly and in well-ventilated areas.

Symptoms from "the flu" to headaches have been associated with products we use to clean our furniture, bathrooms and clothes, as well as air fresheners to keep our bathrooms smelling pleasant. Debra Lynn Dadd, in *Nontoxic and Natural,* wrote about a fifteen-year study of housewives in Oregon. *Women who stayed home all day had a 54 percent higher death rate from cancer than women who worked away from home.* The study concluded that the higher rate likely was a consequence of exposure to the chemicals in household products. Dadd's book, along with many others, contains formulas for making your own environmentally safe household products.

A Prescription for Toxic Overload

Often, toxic exposure comes from medical and dental offices, from the very professions that you expect would keep you healthy. Whether it is antibiotics in your food, the drug in your inhaler, steroids on your skin, mercury in your mouth, medicines in your stomach or fluoride in your water, the medical and dental industries are significant sources of toxins. In fact, *medical journals acknowledge that prescription drugs are the third leading cause of death in America (after heart disease and cancer).*

As you recall, prescription and over-the-counter drugs "work" by interfering with normal chemical processes in cells. They are designed to suppress symptoms, but do not cure disease. In fact, by interfering with normal cell function, prescription drugs can cause cellular malfunction, which is the same as causing disease. Decisions about which procedures and medicines to choose should be based on knowledge of the toxicity involved. Every molecule you put into your body is going to have an effect, for better or worse. Almost always, prescription and over-the-counter drugs are for the worse.

Furthermore, physicians label many of today's chronic diseases as being of "unknown etiology," a fancy way of saying "we are clueless about the cause." Actually, many new disease conditions can be traced back (either directly or indirectly) to environmental toxins that bioaccumulate in tissues, contribute to toxic overload, disrupt cell chemistry and cause disease.

The Toxic Truths Inside Your Body

Although we are accustomed to thinking about toxins in the outside world, often we forget about the powerful toxins produced within our bodies. The body must eliminate internal toxins to stay healthy.

Under normal, healthy conditions, the body is designed to control those toxins and protect us against harm. Under other circumstances, however, the toxins produced internally can be a serious problem, worse than anything from the outside world. When these internal toxins are produced excessively or cannot be properly detoxified, they build up in the body and cause disease. In almost any chronically ill person, internally generated toxins play a major role.

When toxins are generated in the digestive system (intestinal toxemia), they enter our bloodstream, and if these toxins are present in excess of the liver's ability to detoxify them, they damage cells all over the body. Intestinal toxemia has been associated with AIDS, allergies, asthma, cancer, cardiac arrhythmias, arthritis, eye problems, high blood pressure, mental problems, headaches, various gastrointestinal conditions, senility, skin problems and other diseases. In my own disease process, the internal toxins I was producing were, indeed, a major contributor to my own physical and mental debilitation.

Intestinal toxemia was the "mysterious" ailment plaguing Michael, who had just completed his junior year at Harvard and had gone off to Europe for the summer with friends. As he was traveling around, he began to feel ill, dizzy and fatigued. He went to see a physician in London who prescribed a drug that did not help. Michael saw other physicians in Germany and Switzerland, but he finally returned home—too sick to remain abroad.

A strapping twenty-one-year-old college student should be at the peak of health. Instead, Michael was suffering from debilitating fatigue, he was lightheaded and dizzy, and he had visual disturbances, not to mention various aches and pains. After many thousands of dollars worth of testing (including a brain scan to check for a brain tumor), Michael's physicians were at a loss to explain his condition and referred him to a psychiatrist. Desperately concerned for her son's future and furious with a medical system that was obviously not working, Michael's mother looked for other options; at that point, she called me.

As with any sick person, I knew exactly what was wrong with Michael: his cells were malfunctioning because of a combination of deficiency and toxicity. The question, as always: How to restore his cells to healthy function? I used the six pathways as a guide and eventually discovered that digestive toxins—a critical aspect of the toxin pathway—were the source of Michael's problems.

Digestive toxins are produced in a couple of ways, notably by an abnormal growth of bacteria or yeast in the intestines and by improperly digested food, which putrefies in the digestive system. Intestinal toxemia creates highly poisonous toxins as well as nutritional deficiency. When bad bacteria and yeasts overgrow, they displace the friendly bacteria necessary for producing nutrients such as the B-complex vitamins, vitamin B_{12} and vitamin K. Friendly bacteria also help to obtain the nutrients we need from the food we eat. Intestinal toxemia causes deficiency and toxicity in most of us, to some degree, because of damage from antibiotics.

Michael had acne as a teenager. His dermatologist had prescribed an antibiotic (tetracycline), and Michael had taken this drug every day for years. Antibiotics were developed to kill bacteria. The problem is that helpful bacteria in your intestines (normal intestinal flora) are needed for good health. Years of taking antibiotics destroyed these helpful bacteria in Michael's digestive system. (Even one course of antibiotics can have this effect.) This situation allowed the overgrowth of abnormal intestinal flora and a yeast called *Candida albicans*.

A yeast infection can produce toxic chemicals that absorb into the bloodstream; also, yeast can physically invade and damage the intestinal tissue in a way that allows other inappropriate materials (undigested food particles, toxic wastes and yeast byproducts) to pass directly into the bloodstream. This condition floods the body with dangerous toxins and allergens, causing food allergies and disrupting the immune system. Some of these toxins are neurotoxic (causing damage to the brain and the nervous system) and may produce symptoms such as fatigue, headaches, apathy, depression, anxiety, mood swings and memory lapses. Intestinal yeast infections also impair the absorption of nutrients, which is a separate but equally serious problem. Disrupting the normal ecology of the gut also invites infection by parasites, which further disrupt gut tissue.

In Michael's case, I suspected problems with internally generated digestive toxins, but to know for certain one must measure. I suggested to Michael that he ask his physician to be tested for candida. (Convincing the physician to do the candida test was not easy. Physicians do not generally look for such infections, and his mother had to put considerable pressure on the doctor.) The test did show that Michael had a candida infection, which he was able to get rid of through natural methods such as taking high-quality probiotics and grapefruit seed extract and by reducing dietary sugar (which was "feeding" the yeast problem). Michael, who had been completely disabled by his disease throughout the summer, was able to go back to Harvard in the fall, complete his senior year and graduate.

Problems such as Michael's are common in America because of the excessive antibiotics that our physicians prescribe. While the use of antibiotics is prudent and necessary in very select cases, for the most part antibiotics unnecessarily damage the digestive system and contribute to intestinal toxemia. This toxemia often subjects us to far more toxicity than the original "germ" that the antibiotic was supposed to kill. Unfortunately, almost everybody in America has taken antibiotics at some point; these drugs are a major cause of health problems, including fatigue and allergies. Intestinal toxemia can be provoked in other ways, by medical drugs such as non-steroidal anti-inflammatory drugs (NSAIDs, including aspirin, ibuprofen, naproxen, ketoprofin, etc.) and oral steroids (cortisone pills, birth control pills, etc.).

Maldigestion of food (exacerbated by medical drugs or not) produces toxins inside your body. A mostly cooked and processed food diet lacking critical enzymes is a common contributor, as is poor chewing of food. Low-fiber diets are also problematic. Whatever the cause, undigested food can rot and poison you while still inside you. Carbohydrates ferment, fats turn rancid and proteins putrefy. The most common symptoms are bloating, constipation, gas, halitosis, heartburn, eye problems, neurological problems and headaches.

Keep protein consumption moderate; diets high in protein, especially cooked meat and pasteurized dairy, overload our digestive systems. We need only 35 to 40 grams of protein per day (more for athletes or those with large body frames), but Americans eat an average of 90 grams of gut-putrefying protein per day. A one-pound slab of roast beef contains more than 100 grams of protein. Large quantities of cooked and denatured proteins, which are harder to digest, can cause an overgrowth of a type of putrefactive bacteria that thrive when food is rotting in the gut. These bacteria produce toxic chemicals such as indole, skatole, phenol and hydrogen sulfide. In addition, these putrefactive bacteria displace friendly bacteria, which are essential to good digestion and health, and the result is intestinal toxemia.

To prevent or eliminate the problems associated with intestinal toxemia:

- Avoid the use of antibiotics, anti-inflammatories and steroids (including birth control pills).
- Avoid excessive amounts of protein.
- Minimize or eliminate processed foods. Eat the right kinds of fats.
- Avoid sugar, white flour, coffee, excessive alcohol and fried foods. These substances are hard on the digestive system.
- Adhere to proper food combining and chewing; the digestion process must begin in the mouth and in the stomach for the intestines to function properly.

Do you suffer from indigestion, bloating, gas, cramping, loose stools, constipation or gastrointestinal reflux? Any of these can indicate intestinal toxemia and should be addressed before they lead to serious disease.

You can also consider other strategies if you are suffering from symptoms of poor digestion: fasting, exercising, drinking large amounts of water, and taking high-quality supplements, including probiotics, digestive enzymes, and vitamins and minerals. All of these help to detoxify, repair and rebuild healthy tissue—in particular by helping to create an environment in the digestive system conducive to the growth and maintenance of friendly bacteria.

Allergies Should Signal Alarm

Allergies are a common source of internally generated toxins. Every allergic reaction produces metabolic debris that
has a toxic effect. We tend to think of allergies as "normal," a
benign inconvenience, because so many people have them.
Not so. Healthy people do not have allergies. Allergies are an
abnormal immune response to foods and substances in your
environment. Most food allergies are the result of an abnormally functioning digestive system, as already mentioned,
whereby undigested food molecules are allowed to enter the
bloodstream though damaged gut tissue. The immune system recognizes these food particles as foreign, and you have
an immune response called an allergy. The body remembers
this response; every time you eat the offending food, an
allergic reaction—and the toxins created by that reaction—
is produced.

When an offending substance, called an allergen, reacts
with an antibody produced by the immune system, large
amounts of allergen/antibody (immune) complexes can be
formed. If immune complexes are formed in greater quantities
than the body can handle, they can be deposited in tissues
(such as brain arteries, brain membranes, small blood vessels,
the liver, the uterus, the lungs and the kidneys), where they are
capable of clogging blood vessels and joints and are known to
release chemicals that cause a cascade of health-damaging
reactions. Through this mechanism, immune complexes may
be responsible for up to 90 percent of all kidney disease.

*Allergies are an indication of systemic illness and should be
considered a serious immune dysfunction disease.* If you are
allergic (and most Americans have allergies and intolerances,
although they may be unaware of it), determine the substances
you react to and avoid them. More importantly, strengthen
your immune system, through diet and supplements, so these
reactions will not occur in the first place; optimize your

body's ability to detoxify so that you can minimize damage caused by the allergic reactions you do suffer.

Stress Poisons in Many Ways

Stress can be loosely defined as any demand we place upon the body; the body's reaction to these demands causes us to "feel stressed." Everybody knows that stress is hard on us, but few people understand why, on a physical level. Chronic stress literally poisons you.

The body's response to stress—often called the "fight-or-flight response"—refers to feelings of anger or fear that generate the release of chemicals in your body, designed to give you more strength in an emergency.

In an emergency situation that passes quickly—for example, you rush to catch someone who is falling—the body is able to detoxify the stress chemicals that are produced. However, when stress is chronic, and we constantly live our lives in stressful ways, these chemicals build up and inflict damage to our cells. Common stress symptoms include muscle wasting, fatigue, osteoporosis, high blood pressure, fragile blood vessels, suppressed immunity, impaired mental function and a host of other problems. What stress is, how it affects you (physically and psychologically) and what you can do about it will be explored more in chapter 7, which explores the psychological pathway.

As we have discussed, the cells in your body naturally produce toxic byproducts that a healthy body is designed to handle. If the body becomes overloaded with toxins, for whatever reason, even normal metabolic toxins can add to the total toxic load and damage cells. Chronic, internally generated stress chemicals can often move us into toxic overload.

Illnesses also stress us with massive amounts of internally generated toxins, which is why we must choose health in the first place. When symptoms of illness do manifest, cells are malfunctioning and the body is struggling desperately to make itself well again. Under these extra stress loads, to minimize the damage done, taking steps to optimize cellular function becomes even more important.

Your Primary Toxic Defense: The Liver

Various organs in the body—kidneys, bowels, lungs, lymph system and the skin—are designed to eliminate metabolic waste. Fiber helps "carry out the garbage" in the digestive system, and exercise helps us detoxify via sweating and movement of the lymphatic system. Water promotes detoxification through the kidneys and sweat glands, and saunas assist in removal of both water and oil-soluble toxins.

At any given time, about 25 percent of all the blood in your body is in your liver, awaiting detoxification. This process begins with a sophisticated filtering system that captures and digests foreign debris. Next, enzymes, produced by the liver, deactivate and eliminate toxins. If these enzymes are interfered with—either deactivated by environmental toxins such as lead and mercury or never manufactured in the first place because of nutrient deficiency—toxic overload is certain to result. Liver enzyme detoxification has two phases: In phase one, the liver produces enzymes that take harmful toxins such as alcohol, pesticides, herbicides and prescription drugs, and oxidizes them (burns them) in preparation for removal from the body. This process creates potentially harmful free radicals that must be neutralized with dietary antioxidant nutrients. In phase two, more enzymes are used to combine the oxidized chemicals from phase one with other molecules, which then can be excreted harmlessly in the bile or urine. In both phases, the food we eat supplies the raw materials needed to produce all of these enzymes and other chemicals that are required. These elegant detoxification systems depend on a constant supply of nutrients, which we must obtain from our diet, but we frequently do not.

Help your liver's phase-one detoxification process with antioxidant nutrients: vitamins C, E and A, along with coenzyme Q10, carotenoids, bioflavonoids, selenium, manganese, copper and zinc. Some of these nutrients neutralize free radicals directly; others activate enzymes that neutralize them. Red, yellow and green vegetables are loaded with these antioxidant nutrients. Assist your liver's phase-two detoxification with cruciferous vegetables, such as cabbage, broccoli, cauliflower, green onions, kale and brussels sprouts. These vegetables enable the liver to eliminate powerful carcinogens, helping to protect us against cancer. These dietary suggestions, combined with high-quality supplements, can keep your liver's toxic defenses at peak function.

Much of our body is made of water; the kidneys need it to excrete water-soluble toxins. Water constantly moves throughout your body and must be changed frequently to keep it pure. A minimum of eight glasses of pure water should be consumed every day, and more is better. Your water supply must be pure so as not to add to your toxic load. Water should be consumed as water, not as beverages such as coffee, tea or alcohol (these substances may cause the body to lose water). Water is a simple choice, often overlooked. Dehydration is a common problem, especially among our elderly population.

A toxic lifestyle is often created unwittingly. We fail to appreciate that many small toxic exposures over time, to a wide variety of toxins, lead to an accumulation, causing our cells to malfunction. Even small amounts of toxins can perform amazing feats of chemistry by inhibiting hormones, deactivating enzymes, compromising our detoxification systems and using up precious nutrients. Toxicity is seldom recognized as a primary cause of our health problems. The toxic invaders in our lives—whether they are brought into our homes or they are created in our own bodies—are also not easily detected by typical "radar." The toxins that harm us seldom are labeled hazardous, and they are difficult to identify.

Once we understand the role toxins play in cellular malfunction, we can understand the importance of minimizing toxic exposure and maximizing the body's ability to detoxify. In order to protect yourself and your family, you must learn how to spot these silent and hidden dangers, and how to keep your defenses strong in order to avoid toxic overload. Never before has the human body been faced with such challenges of personal and global pollution. To respond to these challenges and to move yourself in the right direction on the toxin pathway, learn to make the daily choices that will reduce your toxic exposure and support your detoxification systems.

7

THE PSYCHOLOGICAL PATHWAY

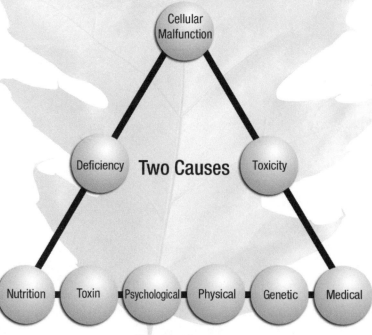

One Disease

Cellular Malfunction

Deficiency   Two Causes   Toxicity

Nutrition   Toxin   Psychological   Physical   Genetic   Medical

Six Pathways

"The simple truth is, happy people generally don't get sick. One's attitude toward oneself is the single most important factor in healing or staying well. Those who are at peace with themselves and their immediate surroundings have far fewer serious illnesses than those who are not."

Bernie Siegel, M.D.
Love, Medicine & Miracles

Even when nutrients are scarce and toxins abundant, one's potential for health is nearly limitless, and it relies almost entirely on ourselves and the power of the mind. Thoughts and emotions have a tremendous effect on our cells and therefore our health. What we put into our minds may be more important than what we put into our bodies. The power of the mind is your best ally in choosing to get well and stay well. *You are what you think.*

"How can it be," you might ask, "that the mind has so much control over the body?" This question assumes that one is separate from the other; in fact, they are inseparable. All the cells in our body contribute to what we call the mind, and what goes on in our mind affects what happens in all our cells.

Chemical reactions are produced throughout the body by

our thoughts, emotions and interactions with others. Fear makes us turn pale; embarrassment makes us blush. Modern science has proven that these "thought chemicals" either can be beneficial or detrimental to health. *We can choose what we put into our minds, and in doing so, we can choose between health and disease.*

This concept is sometimes difficult for people to embrace because thought chemicals are abstract. Their effect, though, is reflected in Dr. Bernie Siegel's 1986 book, *Love, Medicine & Miracles*: "If I told patients to raise their blood levels of immune globulins or killer T-cells, no one would know how. But if I can teach them to love themselves and others fully, the same change happens automatically."

Consider how thought chemicals can improve or damage health:

- A 1991 study in the *New England Journal of Medicine* found that stressful life situations (such as losing a job, breaking off an engagement or simply feeling over-whelmed by life's problems) nearly doubles the risk of catching a cold.
- A thirty-five-year study (1946–1981) of Harvard graduates showed that people who had a pessimistic outlook on life suffered significantly more disease after age forty-five than people with a positive outlook.
- A 2001 study in *Psychosomatic Medicine* found that optimism protects against heart disease. People who are pessimistic and blame themselves for everything were much more likely to die of a heart attack than their optimistic counterparts.
- Dr. O. Carl Simonton, in his 1978 book, *Getting Well Again,* talks about how visual imagery with positive mental images had a beneficial effect on patients with advanced cancer. Simonton found that people who used their minds to heal had double the survival rate of those who did not.

- A study in a 2000 issue of *Lancet* concluded that women who experience severe emotional stress during the first trimester of pregnancy are 80 percent more likely to have a child with birth defects.

Body, Heal Thyself

You must believe in your health if you are to maintain or regain health. You must actively care for your health when you are well, and actively pursue wellness when you are ill.

When my own body was in progressive deterioration during the depths of my illness, I began to realize that, for survival, I needed to employ my mind as well as my body. I began to repeat a version of an old affirmation to myself, again and again, a mantra of sorts: *Every day, in every way, I get stronger and stronger and better and better.*

At first, when I would say this to myself, my mind would fight back, saying something like, *Wow, are you a liar! You feel worse today than you did yesterday.* I realized that my positive mental affirmations were being negated by my own thinking about my situation. I began to reply to my mind's objections by saying, *I know I am worse today, but I am giving you an instruction.*

Once I became comfortable giving my body instructions, my own objections began to disappear and my body began to respond. I would say my affirmation, sometimes out loud, with passion and expectancy, many times daily, repeatedly, until I could feel strength coming into my body as I said the words. After a few weeks, my subconscious mind began to implement the instructions and intent of my conscious mind. One day, after saying these affirmations, I felt the best that I had felt since the onset of my illness. The feeling lasted only five or ten minutes, but the fact that it happened proved that I was on the right path. Soon, the feelings of strength came more often and lasted longer. Later in my studies, I learned of the close connection between the mind and the immune system. My badly damaged immune system was responding!

These affirmations had a profound effect on me. I began to understand that health and disease can be the reactions of the subconscious mind to the thoughts of the conscious mind; the subconscious takes orders from the conscious mind and implements them. Minds do what they are programmed to do, even though much of that programming is unintended. I began to realize my power to influence my health simply by choosing the daily thoughts I was putting into my mind. By focusing on my illness, I had been putting thoughts of disease into my mind, thereby creating more disease. The mind is always working, so why not make it work for rather than against you? Keep your images and suggestions as positive, simple, clear and concise as possible. Then repeat them as often as possible. Allow the subconscious to accept them as a command and implement them.

Over the past sixteen years, of all of the people I have known with "incurable" and "fatal" diseases, the thrivers and survivors have been those individuals who used the power of their minds to heal their bodies consciously. Take the case of Karl, a concert violinist who became paralyzed by a stroke. His physicians told him the paralysis was permanent. Confined to a wheelchair, Karl was unwilling to accept such a fate. He decided to use the power of his mind to establish new connections in his brain. He started by focusing intensely on just one finger. He commanded it to move, and eventually it did! Now a medical curiosity, in 2001 Karl was invited to give a concert at an international medical conference where his doctor presented his story. Brain scans show that Karl's miraculous recovery resulted from using entirely new areas of his brain and bypassing the damaged areas. Music critics claim he is playing better than ever! How's that for the power of the mind?

Choosing to Stay Sick

In contrast to Karl, other people in my experience have failed to strengthen their psychological pathway and lost the health benefits of positive efforts. Lisa was one. She had suffered from extreme chemical sensitivity for twelve years before coming to me for help. I was confident I could help her, based on my own experiences. I taught Lisa how to improve her health, mostly through dietary and vitamin supplement suggestions, and she made some striking initial improvements. After a few months, Lisa was living her life in ways that she had not been able to for many years; she had started dating, going out dancing and even going on sailing trips. Lisa's friends commented about how well she looked and her good progress. After twelve years of sickness, Lisa seemed to be on a path to a more meaningful life. She learned what was necessary to choose health and seemed to have developed the psychological willingness to stick with it.

One day, I received a frantic call from Lisa. Her disability caseworker had contacted her and informed Lisa that it was time for an annual review. Lisa had been receiving disability funds from social security and state welfare, and she was living in subsidized housing. For many years, Lisa had been too sick to work and needed this financial support. Now, her health having taken a dramatic turn for the better, Lisa feared that her caseworker would notice the improvement and revoke financial assistance. Lisa panicked.

She had been unable to work for so many years that she had not a clue about how she could support herself without those benefits. Perhaps her desire to get well simply could not compete with her fear of losing support. Perhaps twelve years of "sickness programming" deprived Lisa of the self-confidence she needed to thrive. Sadly, the last time I heard about her, Lisa had stopped applying what she had learned about deficiency and toxicity, and her health had regressed. The potential to get well (that is, her new diet, supplements and workout program) was lost because she could not unlearn her programming to be dependent and disabled.

Will You Care for Me If I Am Well?

Unhealthy psychological programming derailed the health efforts of another client named Ruth, who suffered from chronic fatigue syndrome. Although she followed my recommendations regarding diet and nutritional supplements, she made only modest improvement, and I realized that Ruth was going to be a tough case. I suspected that she needed a great deal of assistance along her psychological pathway.

I learned that when Ruth was a small child, the only time her father paid attention to her was when she was sick. Then, he would buy her toys, sit by her bed and read her stories. Most other times, he either ignored her or related to her superficially. Subconsciously, Ruth learned, "If I want attention, I need to be sick." No doubt she did not intend this, but her behavior was programmed nevertheless. Years later, when her marriage was falling apart and her husband was giving his attention to someone else, Ruth's programmed response was to get sick—this time in order to regain the attention and affection of her husband. In the long run, of course, this kind of behavioral pattern inevitably fails; Ruth's husband eventually divorced her, leaving her alone and sick.

For Lisa and Ruth, certain "rewards" for being sick superseded their desires to get well or stay well. This way of life is not uncommon; people often have psychological reasons to get sick or stay sick—usually not on a conscious level. People often learn hopelessness instead of hopefulness.

If you are sick, be sure to ask yourself, *What is my reward for being sick? Am I willing to give up my reward? Do I truly want to be well?* These questions can be followed with affirmations or mantras, such as *I am well. I am getting better, healthier and stronger every day.* Reprogramming your mind-set or approach is the key, whether you are talking about the thoughts you think or the foods you eat. Health is a choice, and the best chance to realize it comes from making your top priority to get well and stay well.

The Placebo Effect

One of the most familiar descriptions of the power of the mind over the body's responses is the placebo effect. This concept is based on research by Henry K. Beecher, published in a 1955 paper, "The Powerful Placebo," which concluded that roughly one-third of people who receive medical treatment will show improvement simply because they believe the treatment will work, regardless of how pharmacologically effective the treatment is. People's thoughts affect their health—not exactly a news flash, but a scientific fact nevertheless. When the research was published, Beecher's paper made a huge impact on the scientific community, and since then, thousands of published studies on the same topic demonstrate clearly that what you think affects how your body functions.

The term placebo refers to a substance, procedure or treatment that, when given to a patient, produces a beneficial effect on the body that is not a direct result of the placebo's chemistry. Now, medical scientists use placebos to measure the effectiveness of a certain treatment—often a medication—versus "no treatment" at all. In a typical study, for instance, one group of patients is given a drug and another group of patients, unknown to them, receive pills that contain essentially nothing—a placebo.

This approach and the results based on this approach, however, are misguided because the placebo—by virtue of positive thinking—does have effects. Doctors and scientists portray their disrespect for the patient's power by thinking of the placebo as something to be "factored out of the equation," as an unwanted, or at best, uninteresting effect. More medical support for this power could go a long way toward helping all become and stay well.

Scientific work with the placebo proves what we already know instinctively: Beliefs, attitudes and patterns of behavior play a major role in health and disease. Our state of mind is as much a part of our lifestyle as our diet, amount of sleep or exercise. Let us harness the principles of the placebo effect and use that power. In a sincere, direct and informed manner, we can use it more profoundly.

The Best Health Coverage

The support, encouragement and good bedside manner of a health practitioner (be it a modern practitioner or an ancient witch doctor) can help a patient recover, even if this "help" exists only through the "effect of the mind."

Down through history, many or perhaps most of the successes of health-care treatments have been and are due to behavioral and psychological factors. A 1993 study in *Cardiology* raised the possibility that a large share of the presumed benefits of prescription drugs actually results from people believing they are being helped.

New York Times columnist Margaret Talbot summed up this idea, noting that "the truth is that the placebo effect is huge." In studies of new drugs, she says, between 35 and 75 percent of patients benefit from taking a dummy pill. This "placebo effect," she writes, "should probably be put to conscious use in clinical practice, even if we do not entirely understand how it works."

Talbot continues:

For centuries, Western medicine consisted of almost nothing but the placebo effect. The patient who got better after a bleeding—or a dose of fox lung, wood lice, tartar emetic or any of the other charming staples of the 19th-century pharmacopoeia—got better either in spite of them or because of their symbolic value. Such patients believed in the cure and in the authority of the bewigged gentlemen administering it, and the belief gave them hope and the hope helped make them well. There were exceptions—remedies, like quinine for malaria, the vaccine for smallpox and morphine for pain relief, which actually worked. But generally speaking, if all the drugs of the day "could be sunk to the bottom of the sea," as Oliver Wendell Holmes observed in 1860, "it would be all the better for mankind—and all the worse for the fishes."

We need to use the principles of the placebo effect deliberately—without trying to deceive the patient—to benefit health and performance. Imagine the potential gains if modern health care included an educational and "coaching" dimension as part of a more comprehensive approach to healing. This rarely happens. Modern health care focuses almost exclusively on diagnosing and treating the physical body, usually with drugs or surgery, and typically fails to consider the behavioral, emotional, perceptual, learning, cognitive and spiritual factors that may be playing a significant role in becoming sick or well.

Believing that you "have" a disease and playing the role of a "sick person" is the way to stay sick. By contrast, being healthy means believing that you are getting well and staying well; it means "playing the role" of health. *Every thought has a physical effect on your cells.* Negative thoughts, particularly about disease and death, can literally kill you.

An Infection of Negative Thoughts

Although we used to think of mind and body as entirely separate, the last twenty-five years of scientific research have taught us a great deal about the dimensions of mind and body and how, together, they establish body-wide communication networks. Our bodies create chemical messengers (neuropeptides, neurotransmitters and hormones) that allow the body to communicate with itself, to self-regulate, to adapt. Through these chemical messengers the cells know when and what to do. Cells throughout the body (not just in the brain) both create and are affected by these chemical messengers. All cells are in constant contact with one another, whether they are brain cells, muscle cells, nerve cells or any other kind.

Every thought and emotion triggers the release of chemical messengers throughout the body; in other words, there is no such thing as "just a thought." Every thought has a physical consequence, for better or worse. Feelings of anger, apathy, gloom and resentment weaken the immune system and damage health. Positive thoughts of love, compassion, joy, humor and the like support good physical health.

It takes some effort and discipline, especially on the bad days, to keep an open and positive mindset, but the health benefits definitely make it worthwhile. The goal of this chapter is to explain how psychology affects health at the cellular level and to identify some of the most important psychological concepts, as well as some of the most common (and self-destructive) mistakes. The goal is to help you improve your psychological pathway—one of the major avenues between health and disease.

Minds Need Reprogramming

Our minds are rather like computers: Whether intended or unintended, they do what they have been programmed to do. A big part of using the psychological pathway to stay healthy is the ability to recognize your current programming and to learn new programs—new thoughts, attitudes and behavior patterns.

As demonstrated by my clients Lisa and Ruth, some people

find it hard to develop the will to change old patterns. For these two women, habitual thinking and imagery created their destiny. They were in reach of health, but let it go. Why? Not because they lacked the necessary information, the problem most people face, but because their strategies for achieving short-term security had been tried and proven, and were too difficult to unlearn.

Negative health programming can come from a visit to the doctor. Even the sight of a physician can cause blood pressure to rise; the effect is called "white-coat hypertension." The stress resulting from the diagnosis of a grave disease can do serious damage, precisely like voodoo or a witch's hex. A 1991 study in the *Medical Journal of Australia* concluded that negative suggestions from physicians and caregivers were significant negative factors in cancer recovery. Deepak Chopra, M.D., made a similar observation in his book, *Creating Health:* "I have frequently observed that a rapid progression of symptoms and then death from cancer occurred *after* the diagnosis of cancer was made. It is almost as if the patient was dying from the diagnosis and not from the disease."

Physicians must exercise great care not to create negative expectations. We need support and reassurance from our physicians and caregivers. We need them to believe in us and to help us through our processes of healing and recovery. Certainly, we expect honesty from them, but we do not need discouraging remarks and ominous statistics about our slim chances for survival (as I was told that nothing more could be done for me, before I saved my own life).

Regardless of what your health practitioner says or does, getting well and staying well is your responsibility. Taking that responsibility actually helps make you healthier. Unfortunately, most patients relinquish this responsibility to their doctor. They play a passive role of bystander or victim; they think of the health-care provider as their problem solver.

Patients' positive attitudes toward their health or disease

help to make them not only informed but also empowered. Approaching health care with the belief that you, as the patient, are in charge can vitalize your efforts. You ask more questions. You feel more control over the outcome. As Bernie Siegel, M.D., reminds us in *Love, Medicine & Miracles,* the patient must be the primary source of healing. "Exceptional patients," he wrote, "refuse to be victims. They educate themselves and become specialists in their own care. They question the doctor because they want to understand their treatment and participate in it. They demand dignity, personhood, and control, no matter what the course of disease."

There is nothing wrong with going to the doctor—so long as you realize that your health is your responsibility, not your doctor's or anyone else's. Because belief in your own health makes a critical difference, you need to work with professionals who acknowledge how essential this outlook is. You need caregivers to support you in your efforts to participate, and who can assist you in educating yourself productively, rather than hinder you, which is often the case.

Often, psychological healing is thought to be unimportant to treatment in modern health care, but the miracle is precisely the opposite. Unfortunately, modern medicine overlooks the whole person. "Fixing" only the physical body, as if it were a separate entity, is to overlook the complex weave of physiological, psychological and spiritual dimensions that define human beings—including you, your tissues and all of your cells. The standard approach is not good enough.

Healthy Mind, Healthy Immune System

Negative behaviors, thoughts, emotions and stress can adversely affect the functioning of your immune system; they can lower your resistance to infections and make you more susceptible to bacteria, fungi, viruses and other microorganisms. Yet, you can exercise control. You can begin immediately, actively and consciously to improve your ability to fight disease and maintain optimal health.

Speaking about the psychological dimension of the immune system, David Felton, M.D., professor of neurobiology and anatomy at the University School of Rochester, said, "Now there's overwhelming evidence that hormones and neurotransmitters can influence the activities of the immune system and that products of the immune system influence the brain."

In order to protect you from infections, your brain and your immune system must be in constant dialogue. The brain sends information to the immune system by producing certain types of chemical messengers (neuropeptides). That information is delivered to immune cells through receptor sites on cell membranes. Rather like plugging an electrical appliance into a wall outlet, chemical messengers from your brain "plug in" to the receptor sites on the immune cells. This messaging process happens on a very large scale, allowing the brain to deliver information to immune cells throughout the body. Likewise, the body's immune cells respond by creating new chemical messengers, sending information back to the brain. This process creates a constant link or feedback loop between the brain and the immune system.

The role of the psychological pathway in immune system function is illustrated by a study of twenty-six bereaved spouses. The study demonstrated that the pain and stress of bereavement significantly depressed the effectiveness of the immune system. In other studies, depressed immunity in students, determined by the number and activity of T-cells, has been shown to result from the psychological stress of taking exams. Psychologically depressed immunity can even lead to cancer. As far back as the second-century A.D., the physician and philosopher Galen observed that melancholy dispositions disposed women toward developing breast cancer. A 1998 study in the *Journal of the National Cancer Institute* came to the same conclusion. In that study, women who experienced long-term depression were almost 90 percent more likely to develop cancer than their upbeat counterparts.

The Jekyll and Hyde of Stress

Stress has an upside and a downside. Stress can induce positive emotions—excitement, passion and positive arousal. Alternatively, stress can bring on negative emotions such as fear, anxiety and anger. In both cases, the same body systems are involved; both "good" excitement and "bad" fear can increase heart rate and blood pressure. With different mental outlooks, however, different results occur. In a positive mental outlook, health improves; with a negative mindset, cells are damaged and health is impaired. Meeting the stressful challenges that appear in our lives—the chance for a promotion at work, for instance—can help us to grow and develop. When chronic and negative, however, stress damages our cells and impairs our health.

Any perceived threat, such as an attacking predator, a crazy driver or an urgent deadline, causes your nervous system to stimulate both the pituitary and the adrenal glands, releasing stress hormones such as adrenaline. These hormones provide a "rush" necessary to prepare the body for sudden action—by increasing heart rate, breathing rate, blood flow to the muscles, blood pressure and other vital functions. This stress reaction was historically important for survival—part of the "fight or flight" response, which enables us to enhance performance through an increase in our physical and mental capacities for an immediate shift into "emergency mode."

Production of these chemicals, however, was meant to be episodic; an emergency would come, and it would pass. Unfortunately for many people, stress is now chronic. People are working more and sleeping less, and the pace of daily living is accelerating. When chronically mobilized, stress chemicals build up in our system and damage our cells and tissues.

Stress chemicals can lead to damaged immunity, increased susceptibility to infectious disease, damaged blood vessels, maldigestion, sleep disturbance, water retention, fat deposits, hypoglycemia, ulcers, anxiety, high blood pressure, cardiac irregularities, lower pain threshold, lower sperm count, reduced sexual performance, anxiety and depression.

- According to the Occupational Safety and Health Administration (OSHA), stress is among the top-ten reasons Americans miss work.
- The American Medical Association (AMA) has estimated that up to 70 percent of all patients seen by general-practice physicians show symptoms directly related to stress.
- Job stress can chronically raise blood pressure, and stress from lack of control on the job can even increase the risk of heart disease (such as, for example, by changing the parameters of blood clotting factors).
- On a positive note, a 1997 study at Duke University showed that heart attack victims who learned to manage their stress levels could reduce the risk of a repeated heart attack by 74 percent.

Unfortunately, many of us now spend much time during the day in emergency mode as a result of all kinds of what should be nonemergency activities, such as catching buses, driving cars, attending meetings and doing daily work. As a result, we flood our systems with stress chemicals unnecessarily, and we do so on a chronic basis.

To minimize damage from chronic stress, we must find healthful ways to adapt. Adaptation is what stress management is all about. Our ability to adapt is part of what has allowed humankind to survive so well in diverse environments. We must learn how to choose and interpret today's challenges in ways that convert potentially dis-stressful situations to exciting, challenging ones, as well as learn productive coping strategies when dis-stress is unavoidable.

If you know of a certain person, situation or location that stresses you, choose to avoid putting that stress on yourself by avoiding that person, situation or location. Do not put pressure (stress) on yourself when doing so will likely have no effect on the outcome of a situation. You have the power to choose. If you are stuck in a traffic jam, you can either stress out, or you can seize the opportunity to breathe deeply and relax. Neither action makes the traffic move faster, but one approach makes you healthier and the other makes you sicker. If you become visibly irritated when standing in lines or following slow drivers, at those times you may want to evaluate the degree to which you allow life's little irritations to impact negatively on your health and well-being.

Many dis-stressful situations are impossible to avoid. In fact, we would not want to avoid all of them. As Robert Ornstein, M.D., and David Sobel, Ph.D., explain in their book *The Healing Brain,* "If we . . . tried to avoid [all] stressors no one would ever marry, have children, take a job, get divorced, or invent anything at all." "The way we react to stress," they say, "appears to be more important than the stress itself. . . . [T]he onset and course of disease are strongly linked to a person's ability and willingness to cope with stress. . . . Helplessness is worse than stress itself."

Many effective techniques exist for reducing the stress in our lives, including counseling, prayer, meditation, therapy, exercise, yoga, self-hypnosis, keeping a journal, social support and other alternatives. Find what works for you and understand that your health is constantly affected by the way you respond to and interpret the stressful situations in your life; your levels of dis-stress are determined by your choices, not simply by the random happenings in your busy life.

Love Leads the Way

The "good" emotions—love, compassion, spiritual aware-ness—have extremely powerful implications for health, but they are often difficult to define, explain or measure. These complex and nontangible concepts remain perhaps the most "real" considerations in our lives. Understanding their power over health and disease is critical to understanding and prac-ticing effective health care.

Strong social support—including family relationships, friendships, relationships with health practitioners, romantic relationships, and relationships with spiritual leaders and fig-ures—is a critical component of health care. People are typi-cally healthier and recover from diseases more effectively when they have strong social ties. Why? Perhaps people simply feel cared for and hopeful about their future. Or per-haps the bonds that people form transcend our traditional sci-entific understanding of health—even into realms of spirit and energy. However it works, people who relate with others do help each other through adversities, allowing for greater health and wellness than people who are isolated and alone.

Although relationships cannot be put onto a slide and exam-ined under a microscope, many studies have cited the effects of relationships—or the lack of relationships—on health and disease:

- People who are single, separated, divorced or widowed are more than twice as likely to die than their married peers, and five to ten times more likely to be hospitalized for mental disorders.
- Social isolation is as big a risk factor for disease as smoking.
- People with minimal social connections, such as those with few friends or family and people who tend not to participate in their communities, are two to five times more likely to die prematurely than those with more

extensive social ties. These differences are independent of age, sex, and ethnic or cultural background.

• Studies of medical students during stressful exam periods found that the biggest drop in immunity occurred in students who reported being lonely.

• When experimental subjects were injected with cold viruses, individuals with fewer social ties were four to six times more likely to develop colds as those who had more social ties.

• The death rate among Russian men increased by nearly 40 percent following the fall of communism, attributed to social instability.

Love is a deep and vital part of ourselves and a critical aspect of the psychological pathway. There is love for oneself, for other people, for pets, love in spiritual practice and much more. True love, of course, is unconditional, existing for its own sake because you choose it and want it in your life.

Finding and feeling love, however, can be a challenge. Anger, frustration, fear, jealousy, apathy—all can interfere with our ability to love ourselves and those dear to us. Part of being able to love is being able to have compassion both for yourself and for the people around you. Understanding the obstacles that you face in your life makes it possible and easier to understand the obstacles others face. Within this perspective, you can have compassion for anyone, even someone who mistreats you. Likewise, having compassion for yourself is not only possible but essential! Sometimes we succeed and sometimes we fail; facing life's obstacles is challenging, as we all know, but without compassion and love, obstacles may seem insurmountable.

If we do not fill our lives with love and compassion, then we make room for their opposites, such as anger and hostility, which are incredibly harmful to our health and happiness. As Redford Williams, M.D., author of the book *Anger Kills,* wrote: "Getting angry is like taking a small dose of some slow-acting poison every day of your life." At the Behavioral Medicine Research Center at Duke University, Williams has researched the effects of anger, particularly how stress chemicals cause heart disease. He found that chemicals released by the body during periods of anger and hostility damage the lining of arteries. Another study reported in a 1980 issue of *Psychosomatic Medicine* found that people who are cynical, who have hostile attitudes and who have suppressed anger have more atherosclerosis and blockage of coronary arteries and are more likely to have heart attacks.

The Power of Prayer

Perhaps the best way to maintain love and compassion in your life is to consciously seek and practice it. Enlightened leaders and global spiritual traditions advocate spiritual practice as the essential foundation of comprehensive health and vitality, including all aspects of a sound mind and body. This book does not advocate any specific religion or spiritual practice, but does recommend some type of practice. Why? Because being self-involved, self-centered and "stuck in your own head" is so easy. Only when body, mind and spirit are fully integrated can you truly optimize your health.

Spiritual practice brings about measurable changes in the brain and in overall health. Larry Dossey, M.D., in his book *Healing Words,* described "one of the best kept secrets in medical science": the benefits of prayer. Dr. Dossey defines prayerfulness as "a feeling of love, compassion and empathy toward another," and he explains that prayer is "a powerful and legitimate (if often overlooked) method of healing." Dossey uses an impressive array of evidence to show that prayer can have a positive effect on health. A 1988 study conducted in San Francisco investigated the effects of prayer on the cardiovascular health of 393 coronary-care patients. Unknown to the patients involved, one group was prayed for and the other was not. At the end of the ten-month study, the prayed-for group was five times less likely to require antibiotics and three times less likely to develop a condition in which the lungs fill with fluid. Dr. Dossey's research also found that prayer can have beneficial effects on various living cells and organisms, including mice, chicks, fungi, yeast, bacteria and enzymes. In the October 2001 issue of the *Journal of Reproductive Health,* researchers at Columbia University—expressing great surprise at their own profound findings—announced that when complete strangers prayed for women who went to a fertility clinic, the women had twice the pregnancy rate as women for whom prayers were not given.

How does spirituality influence health and performance, and how do we integrate it into health-care promotion and practice as professionals and as individuals? No one scientifically understands the mechanisms. Nonetheless, the scientific data prove that spirituality does work. Such data pose profound questions. Perhaps these precise questions are the ones we need to be asking in order to develop a more complete understanding of health. Even if we don't have all the answers, we can still benefit from the power of spiritual practice.

A Great Opportunity

While health generally is measured and understood at the physical level, as we have discussed, psychological health and physical health are indivisibly one and the same. What goes on in your mind is also going on in your body, and the good news is that you have a wide menu of practical, productive, self-empowering and exciting options to promote psychological—and, therefore, physical—well-being.

Too many people fall into self-defeating lifestyle patterns. If you want to move yourself in the right direction on the psychological pathway and improve your health for the better, you cannot continue to do the same negative things and expect to obtain different and positive results. Changing one's patterns of behavior, belief, thinking, feeling, perception and physical response is the goal of the psychological pathway. Such changes take practice and commitment.

The first step is to notice and identify the feelings associated with stress, then to implement strategies consciously to take care of yourself. Beyond mental techniques—such as prayer, biofeedback, therapy, meditation and numerous self-regulation techniques—physical activities also can be helpful, including exercise, breathing techniques, yoga, massage, saunas and hot baths. Understanding how the mind affects the function (or malfunction) of our cells enables us to make the positive choices that enable us to maintain or improve health.

Keeping a healthy outlook is both one of life's great challenges and one of life's great opportunities. Having a purpose, a higher meaning to your life than mere existence, is a critical part of the whole picture of health.

8

THE PHYSICAL PATHWAY

One Disease

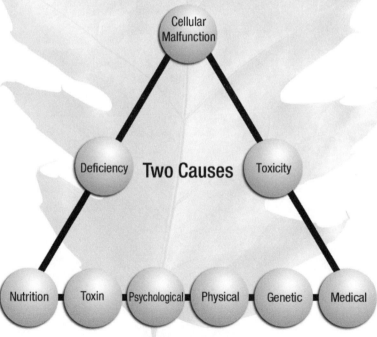

Cellular Malfunction

Two Causes

Deficiency

Toxicity

Nutrition • Toxin • Psychological • Physical • Genetic • Medical

Six Pathways

"Many of the things we call biomarkers of aging might actually be biomarkers of inactivity."

William Evans, Ph.D.
The Human Nutrition Research Center on Aging

Y ou've heard the advice before: If you want to stay physically fit and healthy, get plenty of exercise and sleep, and stay away from drugs, tobacco and alcohol. You may have heard it so often, in fact, that you no longer are paying attention. Also because this advice is common—the kind of thing "your mother told you"—you may think that you know all that you really need to know.

Think again! There is more to the story. Without understanding how everyday choices affect your health at the cellular level, you may not recognize the risks to avoid, nor the benefits you can reap. For example, missing too much sleep may create more than dark circles; it may cause brain damage. Breathing the right way may help you feel better and live longer. Exercising your eyes, in simple ways, may help you to avoid needing eyeglasses, or to discard eyeglasses you already wear. Using hairdryers, electric razors, cellphones and other electrical appliances may increase your risk for cancer, as does exposure to medical X rays. Simple choices can make the difference—turn on the dishwasher only when you plan to leave the kitchen.

- Much of the disability in our elderly population attributed to aging actually is the result of decades of inactivity.
- A study reported in the October 1999 issue of *Lancet* found that after one week of only a few hours sleep per night, hormone levels change and the body even has trouble metabolizing carbohydrates.
- A study reported in the February 2001 issue of *Occupational Medicine* showed that factory workers, chronically exposed to loud noise, suffered calcium and magnesium losses.
- Medical X rays may be the leading cause of cancer.

If you do not support your body's needs for sleep and exercise and protect yourself from physical harm—everything from noise to microwaves to X rays—you cannot be healthy. Also you cannot be overweight and healthy; you cannot be exhausted and well. Terms like "overweight" and "exhausted" are definitions of ill health and, in the long-term, invitations to disaster.

Think of all the people you know: those who wear their age well and those who "break down." Think of all the cars on the streets: beautifully maintained classic cars as well as rusty old "clunkers." If you want long-lasting health, you must maintain your body properly and "drive" it with care.

Maintaining yourself on the physical pathway is not only about preventive maintenance but also about protecting your body from the physical damage that results from physical events (accidents, sport injuries), the environment (noise, sunburn, electromagnetic radiation) and medical treatments (X rays, drugs, surgery).

Given the lifestyles of many Americans who spend most of their days sitting or driving, who have hectic schedules and interrupted sleep and whose days may be bombarded by unrecognized environmental assaults, the time has come to be serious about preventing wear and tear.

The Joy of Movement

Throughout human evolution, our biological ancestors were very active, engaging in hours of vigorous physical activity every day. They walked or ran everywhere they went, and they needed to work hard, physically, to meet their basic needs. Because of this evolutionary history, human bodies require physical activity for good health. Historically, healthy populations such as the Hunzas and the Vilcabambas met those biological needs by default. They lived their entire lives in mountainous farming communities where they had vigorous exercise through regular daily activities. As you recall, older Hunza men—often well into their hundreds—worked in the fields and participated in strenuous folk dancing. *Exercise is like an essential nutrient; without it, your body malfunctions.*

Unlike our hunter-gatherer ancestors, most of us now engage in little physical activity. The Industrial Revolution radically changed human existence. Machines and technology perform work formerly done by hand. No longer do we hunt or farm; our work is done sitting at a desk or standing behind a counter, and we meet our daily needs with a quick trip to a store. Even our recreation is sedentary: We read books, play video games, and watch movies and television (the average American watches three hours a day). We seldom walk or run; instead, we use automobiles, trains, taxis and buses.

Sixty percent of our adult population is sedentary, and one out of four people engages in absolutely no exercise whatsoever. Lack of activity contributes to our epidemic of physical problems such as low-back pain and spine problems, fatigue, arthritis, osteoporosis, obesity and a host of chronic diseases. Almost everyone has the nagging sense that they "should" exercise, but few understand why exercise is so important.

Exercise is good because (like anything else that is "good for you"), it promotes the health of cells. Exercise prevents both of the two causes of disease—deficiency and toxicity—by promoting efficient nutrient delivery to cells and stimulating the lymphatic system (the body's sewage system), vital for removing toxins from cells.

Exercise is great for body and mind; it slows the effects of aging, reduces pain and helps to improve mood, clarity of mind, balance, coordination and spatial awareness—not to mention the confidence boost that comes from "getting physical." The body has almost seven hundred different muscles; without physical activity, these muscles quickly waste away and lose their strength. When certain muscles are weak, others will compensate to do the work, which can cause painful physical damage to the body with long-term wear and tear. What happens then? Canes, walkers and pain medications are the frequently prescribed treatments, but the problem is inactivity. A study reported in the *Journal of the American Medical Association* in 1996 found that physically inactive people are up to twice as likely to die prematurely as those who are physically fit.

Lack of exercise actually may be a greater health risk than smoking. People who exercise regularly and also smoke typically live longer and healthier lives than people who do not smoke but also do not exercise. Consider what happens to bedridden people—bodies that do not move or exercise at all. Their cells become increasingly more deficient and toxic, wasting away daily. Unused muscles lose 10 to 15 percent of their strength per week and half their strength in just three to five weeks. Meanwhile, the bones and joints become weak, brittle and susceptible to fracture or breakage.

Exercise for Your Mind's Sake

Exercise is important for mental function, helping to engage and clear the mind. Lack of exercise makes a person more susceptible to mental illness. Exercise is an excellent stress-management technique. Older people who exercise are 3.5 times less likely to develop Alzheimer's disease than those who lead sedentary lives. Engage in some kind of physical activity every day. Letting days or weeks go by without any exercise has a negative impact on the health of your brain cells as well as all your other cells. The known benefits of exercise include the following:

- Releases brain chemicals that alleviate feelings of anxiety, depression and mental stress.
- Enhances the immune system (by increasing natural killer-cell activity) and improves the body's ability to fight infections.
- Slows the onset of aging effects, such as slowed nerve impulses and bone demineralization (including osteoporosis).
- Reduces the risk of developing Type II diabetes by about 25 percent and decreases insulin resistance.
- Helps lower blood pressure. Regular exercise can lower blood pressure by ten points or more.
- Helps prevent cardiovascular disease by blocking the buildup of plaque in the arteries.
- Dissolves blood clots and reduces the risk of stroke.
- Reduces cancer risk; just four hours of exercise per week lowers a woman's risk of breast cancer by almost 60 percent.
- Tones and conditions the entire body and helps prevent obesity.

Diet Fads and Facts

Dieting to lose weight is a recurring theme in American life. New diet plans are announced repeatedly. Weight-reducing products flood the market, often promoted by famous or ordinary people with "remarkable" stories. For lasting results in any weight-loss program, however, exercise is essential. Decreasing calories (dieting) as a weight-loss method can actually cause the body to slow its metabolic rate to conserve energy. By starving, one has less energy and burns less fat, and the unwanted pounds are likely to stay right where they are. Regular exercise changes how your body produces energy (like stoking a fire or heating up a furnace), increasing one's ability to burn stored fat and lose weight.

America has a serious obesity epidemic that worsens yearly and begins at younger and younger ages. Consider our children, who are spending more time with computers, television and video games, and less time at physical play. From 1960 to 2000, obesity among U.S. children aged six to ten years increased 54 percent. Parents, do not kid yourselves: Few children outgrow weight problems. *Eighty percent of obese children and adolescents become obese adults.* These high obesity levels in children already are contributing to widespread diseases, including cardiovascular disease, diabetes and cancer. These conditions frequently are associated with obesity and used to be rare in children.

The only way to stop this cycle is to start with the kids! At least adults can understand that bodies are made of cells that must be maintained. Young children do not, yet they suffer the repercussions. Adults need to instruct children. We only hurt them when we allow them to develop sedentary and unhealthy lifestyles—when we allow them to sit in front of electronic screens as a way of life, rarely exercising or seeing the light of day.

Gain—Without the Pain

In general, everybody needs some kind of physical movement every day. Establishing and adhering to a routine may be difficult. Realistically, how do you fit a workout into an already busy life? By doing what you like to do. If you do not like a particular type of exercise (and you do it more for the "medicine" than for the enjoyment), you are far less likely to continue it. Experiment until you discover the activity or routine that is right for you, one that genuinely engages you.

A vigorous and challenging exercise routine is ideal, but most importantly, establish a routine that you can practice consistently. Occasional, erratic workouts provide little benefit. Furthermore, intense physical activity with an out-of-shape body increases risk of injury. If you do not exercise every day, absolutely avoid long periods of time (a week or more) of being sedentary; *living a sedentary lifestyle is the same as inviting disease and injury into your body.*

Establishing a healthy exercise routine requires evaluating your body's comfort level and limits. Exercises should be challenging, but not painful. Pain is a warning. Mild discomfort is normal, but once the body is warmed up, pain should go away. If not, perhaps the exercise is too intense, or perhaps more thorough stretching and warmup are needed.

How much exercise do we need? In 1995, the Centers for Disease Control and Prevention and the American College of Sports Medicine surveyed existing evidence. Both organizations recommend that every American get a minimum of thirty minutes of physical activity every day. Within reason, the more intense the exercise, the greater the health benefits. For example, men burning two thousand to three thousand calories per week in their exercise program are 46 percent less likely to experience a stroke than men who burn less than one thousand.

An Exercise Plan That Really Works

Three basic parts of a healthy exercise routine for everyone
should include:

- *Aerobic* exercise. It gets the body warmed up, the heart
  pumping and the blood circulating. Aerobics include jog-
  ging, speed walking, bicycling and fitness classes.
  Aerobic exercise burns fat and calories, maintains fitness
  in the heart and lungs, helps circulate the lymph (thus
  getting rid of toxins) and helps increase the oxygen supplied to bodily tissues (cancer thrives in low-oxygen,
  unexercised tissues). Because it helps prevent both cancer and heart disease, the two biggest killers in America,
  aerobic exercise is probably the most important type of
  exercise.

- *Weight-bearing* exercise. Once the body is warmed up
  (and you've taken time to stretch out and drink fluid),
  weight or resistance training (weightlifting or yoga, for
  instance) is useful to increase muscle strength and
  endurance, as well as to promote healthy bones, joints
  and connective tissues. Such exercise is important in preventing osteoporosis and arthritis. Because of the added
  forces involved in weight-bearing exercise, use of proper
  technique is essential. Poor technique, along with excessive weight or repetition, can cause physical damage.
  Smooth, controlled movements are necessary, as is steady
  breathing (which helps with strength and control).

  The basic weightlifting guideline: three sets of
  weightlifting exercises per muscle group, resting briefly
  between sets, and lifting ten to twenty times per set. Be
  careful not to "jerk" or force exercises, especially if you
  are tired; otherwise you benefit little and are at greater
  risk for injury.

- *Stretching and flexibility.* Before, during and particularly
  after exercise, stretching is important. Rigid, tight tissues

tend be more susceptible to injury, and such tightness also interferes with smooth and efficient joint movements. For these reasons, stretching can help make other aspects of a workout easier and more comfortable. If part of your exercise routine seems unusually challenging or painful, try a brief stretch, which may help you to move with more freedom and comfort. Stretching (again, using steady movements and controlled breathing) makes tissues stronger, healthier and more mobile. This critical aspect of every workout should not be rushed or overlooked.

Determine the specifics of your exercise plan by tailoring it to your own body, and do what you enjoy. Even if you get no other exercise, at least go for a walk each day. Going for a walk (or a hike) can be very pleasurable, and it is good for you. Walking can even provide a good aerobic workout, just by walking faster. The average person strolls along at about three miles per hour. Increasing your walking speed to a brisk stride (about four miles per hour) does a good job working your heart and lungs. Better still, speed walking (about five miles per hour) warms up the body, exercises major muscle groups and actually burns more calories than a slow run of the same speed. For a more complete body workout, consider yoga. Certain types of yoga combine aerobic, weight-bearing and stretching exercises into one complete workout. Many excellent books on yoga are available, and there may be instructional classes available in your local area.

Remember that exercise is supposed to make the body feel better, not worse. The goal is to promote the health of your cells, not to place undue stress on your body.

The intensity of all types of exercise must be moderated. In warmup and aerobics, an extended workout of moderate intensity is preferable to a brief, heart-pounding, sweat-pouring one. Just as a frying pan needs to be warm to cook food, your body needs to be warm for good performance—warm enough to do the job, without "burning." During weight-bearing exercise, build strength and endurance without excessive resistance or repetition. Try holding a weight-bearing pose until the muscles begin to fatigue, then perform the weight-lifting repetitions. Holding prior to repetitions maximizes strength and endurance while minimizing wear and tear.

Your exercise routine should be challenging, but reasonable for individual limits. Avoid approaches such as, "I had better make this a good workout, since I haven't been exercising lately," or "the more strenuously I exercise, the better it will be." During your workout, moderate your intensity by keeping in mind how you will feel afterward. You want to feel like you accomplished a good workout but did not beat yourself up. Consistency, rather than extreme intensity, produces the benefits of exercise. Challenge yourself, but be realistic.

Even for people who hate exercise or think they don't have time to exercise, a simple solution, which I use, is rebounding. Bouncing up and down on a minitrampoline has almost magical effects. The activity is simple, surprisingly easy to do, a lot of fun, safe and can be done by almost anyone regardless of age or physical condition. Rebounding sounds like a panacea, which is what it is! Rebounding tones, conditions, strengthens and heals the entire body, in as little as fifteen minutes per day.

Rebounding is so good for you because it exercises and moves every cell in your entire body. We have always known that exercise is good for health but have never understood why until now: Research presented in 2000 at the annual meeting of the American Thoracic Society found that physically stretching cells has a profound impact on their biochemistry and behavior. Moving and stretching a cell—as rebounding does—helps to supply essential nutrients and to eliminate toxic waste products. When you bounce on a rebounder, your entire body (internal organs, bones, connective tissue and skin) becomes stronger, more flexible and healthier. Both blood circulation and lymphatic drainage are vastly improved.

James White, M.D., of the University of California, San Diego, says that rebounding exercise is "the closest thing to the Fountain of Youth that science has discovered."

Visualize a balloon filled with water. Hold the balloon by its stem and observe how gravity pulls on the water, slightly stretching the balloon. Now, move your hand rapidly up and down and observe how the extra gravitational force causes the balloon to stretch and distort. When you bounce up and down on a rebounder, this effect happens to every cell in your body. Rebounding alternately puts pressure on and takes pressure off body cells, like squeezing a sponge. This moving and stretching of the cells facilitates nutrient delivery and toxin removal, which is exactly what you need to be healthy—without having to go to the gym, work up a sweat, or end up with sore muscles and possible injuries. Rebounding is so efficient because it applies weight and movement to every cell. The extra force of gravity caused by the bouncing strengthens bones and joints, yet without the jarring and potential damage of most impact activities. (For more information on what I selected for my own use, see appendix C.)

Another physical technique is skin brushing. Simply take a natural-bristle bath brush and move it along your skin, up the arms and legs and toward the chest. Doing this activity for a few minutes before taking a bath or shower helps circulate lymphatic fluid and is especially important for people who do not get enough regular exercise.

Good physical fitness is much more than a fashion statement and much more than a way to burn calories and sculpt muscles. Exercise is a fundamental physical need, and you need it every day. What if your job requires sitting at a desk? Sitting for extended periods causes physical health to deteriorate. When sitting for extended periods, take time to stand up and stretch the body (along with relaxing your eyes). Even standing up for a minute or two each hour can make a big difference. Remember, your body is a living, breathing, moving

organism; when you sit motionless for hours on end, meta-
phorically speaking, you begin to die.

Sleep: The Antidrug

Adequate sleep is also a deep physical need and a biological necessity. Adequate sleep is critical for building new cells,
repairing damaged ones and replenishing cellular energy levels. Our lives have become so busy that sometimes we forget
what it feels like to be fully rested and awake. We have forgotten what a good night's rest really is. Busy with the constant call of life's duties, sleep is often pushed aside for more
"pressing" needs. A study by the National Sleep Foundation
found that 64 percent of the adult population does not sleep
the recommended eight hours per night, and 32 percent sleep
less than six hours. To compensate, people use coffee, sugar
and other stimulants, which worsens a bad situation. For some
people, better health can be achieved simply by sleeping
more. Needs are different for each person, some requiring less
sleep than others, and much depends on the quality of the
sleep: whether the sleep is deep and refreshing or fitful and
nonenergizing.

For our biological ancestors, sleeping enough was much
less of a challenge. The sun's rising and setting determined
sleep habits. In centuries past, sleeping was about all you
could do once the sun went down. Only in recent years has the
simple flick of a switch given us light whenever we wanted it.

Now, we live in cities that never sleep. Modern technology
excites and stimulates our lives, and often we find ourselves
awake at all hours of the night. One hundred years ago, people
in developed countries slept nine hours each night. Now, the
average American sleeps about seven, which is insufficient for
most people. Sometimes, people think they can "accomplish
more" if they sleep less. Not so. Being deprived of sleep actually makes people less productive. Furthermore, because the

body repairs and rejuvenates itself during sleep, lack of sleep invites sickness and injury.

Being deprived of adequate sleep for even a few nights dulls the brain, lowers energy levels, increases irritability and depression, and makes people more accident-prone. A Louis Harris and Associates poll found that people who sleep less than eight hours each night often experience problems on the job. Sleep deprivation is a major factor in an estimated one hundred thousand automobile accidents per year. In the short term, sleep deprivation produces unpleasant side effects; long-term, it contributes to cellular malfunction and disease.

Lack of adequate sleep also causes hormone imbalances and interferes with other body functions. A study reported in the October 1999 issue of *Lancet* found that just one week of getting too few hours of sleep per night significantly altered hormone levels and compromised the body's ability to metabolize carbohydrates properly. Chronic disruption of the body's hormone balance invites disease. For example, a potentially harmful hormone called cortisol increases in the brain of an under-rested person. High cortisol levels can damage cells in the brain that control learning and memory. If you are over-tired, take that "spaced-out," forgetful feeling seriously; you may be suffering brain damage. Two other hormones (beneficial ones) normally are produced during sleep and decrease if you are under-rested. One is human growth hormone or HGH, which helps to rebuild tissue. Lack of HGH accelerates the aging process. The other beneficial hormone produced during sleep is prolactin, which governs the immune system. A lack of prolactin can impair immunity. *Sleeping enough and normalizing your sleep patterns help to keep these critical hormones balanced properly.*

Sleep also serves to replenish energy. While asleep, the body creates large amounts of ATP (adenosine triphosphate), a high-energy compound that our cells need, much like a car needs gasoline. If you are tired and cannot sleep enough at night, take a nap—perhaps right after lunch or when you get home from work. Sometimes people avoid napping, because they feel like they are "being lazy." If you lack the energy necessary to do the task at hand, get some rest.

If you have boundless natural energy, consider it a very good sign. How energetic or tired we feel is a good general indicator of how well our bodies are functioning. If you are tired all the time, listen to your body's cry for help. Resting is important, but so is considering how diet, toxic exposure, lack of exercise and other factors affect your overall energy levels. Fatigue is often a symptom of disease—physical, psychological or both. As health improves, fatigue goes away.

Consuming coffee and other stimulants to compensate for fatigue interferes with health and productivity. Even if you do function well on "minimum sleep" (and probably maximum caffeine), long-term damage is still being inflicted, the aging process is being accelerated and probably you are not achieving your optimum potential.

Also, be sure to normalize your sleep pattern. Go to bed and wake up at approximately the same time each day, even on weekends. The body prefers regularity. Before going to bed, avoid caffeine, alcohol and any drugs that may interfere with (or induce) sleep. This practice enables you to sleep naturally and healthily—giving your body the ability to build and repair cells, regulate hormonal balances, and produce the energy you need to do the things you want to do.

Breathing the Right Way

Do not take the breathing process for granted. The body can survive weeks without food and days without water, but only minutes without oxygen. Oxygen is our most vital nutrient, and we obtain it with every breath. The way you breathe can substantially affect how you look and feel, your resistance to disease, and even how long you live. We have control over our breathing; proper breathing technique is an important part of optimizing the physical pathway.

In our society, many people breathe incorrectly—either breathing too much or not enough. Either way, oxygen shortages are produced at the cellular level. Underbreathing (one does not breathe in enough air) is uncommon and usually is the result of serious physical compromise—such as when the lungs are failing. Much more common is overbreathing, called hyperventilation (one breathes too much), which also results in an oxygen shortage at the cellular level. How many people are affected by overbreathing? Almost everyone on occasion, and many people breathe this way chronically.

Overbreathing often is the result of a stressful situation; the stress causes us to breathe too deeply or too quickly, an automatic response preparing us for emergency action. You may recognize this as "panic breathing"—gasping, chest breathing, shallow breathing (panting), irregular breathing, rapid breathing or holding of the breath. On occasion, overbreathing is not a problem, yet the stress of life causes many of us to overbreathe chronically. Numerous side effects are produced, including heart palpitations, irregular heart beat, dizziness, muscle spasms, muscle fatigue, high blood pressure, poor memory, asthma attacks, poor concentration, anxiety, among other symptoms. Overbreathing also causes constriction of the blood vessels to the brain (and heart and elsewhere), resulting in up to a 50 percent reduction of oxygen and glucose to the brain—immediately affecting one's ability to learn, think, remember and perform physically. Little wonder we feel dizzy or lightheaded when stressed.

Breathing too rapidly or too deeply causes the body to lose too much carbon dioxide. Normally, oxygen is transported to tissues by bonding with hemoglobin in red blood cells; carbon dioxide helps the oxygen to "break off" the hemoglobin so that it can be used. Without sufficient carbon dioxide, the oxygen does not break off, tissues become oxygen-deficient, and the result is cellular malfunction and disease. Oxygen deficiency is known to cause cancer. A separate problem, caused by insufficient blood levels of carbon dioxide, is that blood pH can become too alkaline. The body will compensate by dumping out alkaline minerals through the urine, in order to rebalance blood pH. The result is a deficiency of alkaline minerals, such as calcium and magnesium, which contributes to diseases such as osteoporosis.

To breathe correctly, the important step is to bring in air down into the lungs, by using the diaphragm, a deep abdominal muscle that nature intended for breathing. Breathing downward with the diaphragm (belly breathing instead of chest breathing) is an effortless and efficient way to breathe. Unfortunately, people often use their chest and upper back to breathe; chest breathing takes more effort, is less efficient and interferes with normal breathing patterns. Breathing downwards with the diaphragm (as opposed to outwards with the chest) moves the viscera (guts) down and away, making more room for the lungs. This action creates the capacity for more air in your lungs and more oxygen for your tissues, thus enhancing the function of your entire respiratory system, whether you are exercising or at rest. Each breath should begin downwards in the belly, only moving up into the chest when necessary.

Correct breathing should be effortless, through the nose rather than mouth, and relatively slow—at a resting rate of less than fifteen breaths per minute, preferably eight to ten. Here is a simple test to check how you are doing: Lie on your back on the floor, put a book on your abdomen, breathe through your nose, and watch to see if the book goes up and down with each breath. Concentrate on belly breathing until the book moves up and down. Next, count the number of breaths you take per minute. Try to keep breaths per minute at less than fifteen and preferably less than ten. Be careful not to overbreathe. The key word is effortless. Let your body do the breathing for you, as it was designed to do. During aerobic exercise, keep the breath down in the belly and out of the chest as much as possible, and I can almost guarantee that your athletic performance and respiratory health will improve.

Breathing has such profound effects, both physically and psychologically, that many ancient traditions—such as meditation, yoga and martial arts—rely first and foremost on breathing technique.

Damage Control

Maintaining the body is one aspect of the physical pathway; preventing physical damage is the other. Modern life exposes us to many different types of physical damage—from sunburns to car accidents, from kitchen cuts and burns to electromagnetic fields. Some physical hazards of modern life can be avoided, while others cannot. Any time the body suffers damage, though, valuable resources (nutrients) are used to perform repairs. Over time the loss of these nutrients impairs cellular health, opening the door for further injury or disease. Sometimes repair is not possible. Physical damage can lead to lifelong impairment or disability. To prevent damage before it occurs, recognize physical hazards and take sensible precautions. Here are some ways to protect yourself.

Sunbathing Isn't Always a Bad Thing

The body needs sunshine just as it needs food, although one must avoid too much of either. Sunlight (full-spectrum light) is necessary for good health and an important part of the physical pathway. Those warming sun rays feel good because they are good; they help your body produce vitamin D, an essential nutrient for building strong and healthy bones. The common belief that you should protect yourself from the sun with toxic sunscreen is distorted and misguided.

Sunlight is not the problem; the problem is sunburn.

Sunburns only happen from excessive and inconsistent exposure to sunlight, such as when you stay in the sun too long or when your body is not used to it. Regular, controlled exposure to sunlight helps the body produce vitamin D and adapt to the sun. If your body is not used to it (and especially if your skin is fair), do not spend all day under the hot sun. Start out with ten or fifteen minutes of sun per day, gradually increasing your exposure as your body adapts to it. Also, beware of the intensity of the sunlight, when the sun is most directly overhead (approximately 10 A.M. to 2 P.M.).

If you want to protect your skin, using coat after coat of toxic sunscreen is a bad idea. Some of the chemicals in sunscreen can break down when exposed to sunlight, forming carcinogenic compounds. In other words, sunscreen may cause skin cancer, rather than preventing it. Perhaps it is not a coincidence that as sunscreen use has increased, so have skin cancer rates.

Safer alternatives are available to sunburn and toxic sunscreen: Get regular sun exposure, so that your skin can adapt. Dietary nutrients are helpful, including magnesium, antioxidants (vitamins A C, E, selenium), and especially carotenes, which sometimes are referred to as "nature's sun umbrella." Carotenes protect the skin from sunlight; these nutrients are found in colorful vegetables and fruits, such as carrots, sweet potatoes, bell peppers (red, yellow and purple), squash and others. Also, try the ancient custom of rubbing olive oil on the skin to help protect it from sunburn, provided the oil is of high quality and still contains its natural antioxidant chemicals. (Olive oil also is good if your skin is already burned.) People in Mediterranean countries still use olive oil for sun protection today. If you must have a sunscreen, consider one of the toxin-free sunscreens (see appendix C).

Loud Noise Takes a Toll

Ever notice a ringing in your ears after listening to loud music or being around loud noises? That is physical damage, both permanent and cumulative. A study in the January 2001 *Audiology* found that people who engaged in noisy leisure-time activities, ranging from rock concerts to disco dancing to woodworking, have increased risk of hearing loss for each five-year period of participation. Choose to spend your time in less noisy places or wear hearing protection such as earplugs. Hearing loss is now epidemic in America. The hearing aid business grows every year, which is not just a result of the population growing older.

Noise causes other problems, too. Do you ever "jump" when somebody rings the doorbell, when a car alarm goes off, or when the music suddenly is turned louder? In many ways, noise can be stressful, causing both physical and psychological problems. A study in the March 2001 *Journal of the Acoustical Society of America* found that children chronically exposed to transportation noise from road, rail and air traffic had elevated blood pressure and elevated levels of stress chemicals. A similar study in the February 2001 *Psychological Medicine* found that children exposed to chronic aircraft noise have impaired reading comprehension. Noise also causes nutritional deficiency; a study in the February 2001 *Occupational Medicine* measured significant losses of calcium and magnesium in the urine of factory workers chronically exposed to loud noise. Noise studies on laboratory animals have shown other damaging effects, ranging from impaired lymphatic drainage to increased intestinal permeability. A study published in the May 2001 *Behavioral Physiology* concluded that even what we would consider mild chronic noise can cause changes in the lining of the intestines, making them leakier, which can lead to allergies and many other chronic health problems.

While music and other sounds are good for the spirits, avoid living in an environment of never-ending noise. Peace and quiet are great for the psyche. Consider how noise affects you and make your choices accordingly. If you know you are going to be exposed to loud noise, wear ear protection. Diet also helps to prevent hearing loss. Especially if you are genetically predisposed to hearing loss, proper nutrition can have a significant effect on whether such loss will happen or not.

Eye Muscle Exercises Help Save Sight

Most people do not realize the amount of influence they have over their eyesight. Ability to see is greatly dependent on how one uses and exercises their eyes. Like all the muscles in the body, the ones that control eyesight must be exercised in order to keep them supple and strong. Call it "vision maintenance." Modern life requires using the eyes in ways very different from those under which we evolved. Now we must make special choices in order to protect and maintain our natural vision.

The main reason we lose our vision, believe it or not, is literacy. Reading and writing are new skills in the scope of human evolution. During most of human evolution, our eyes were primarily used to gaze afar—to locate food, shelter and threats to safety. When focusing off at a distance, the muscles that control the shape of the eye and the shape of the lens remain in a relatively natural and relaxed state. However, in order to focus on something close, such as a book or a computer screen, the muscles that control the shape of the lens and the eye must contract. For brief periods of time, this reshaping of the eye tissues does not pose a problem. However, we now spend most of our time focusing on nearby objects such as books, papers, televisions and computer screens. We place our eye muscles under constant tension for hours every day, causing a permanent distortion of the lens and the eyeball itself. Thus, vision deteriorates.

To maintain or improve your natural vision, corrective lenses are not the answer. Corrective lenses cause damage to eye tissues, forcing them to work in unnatural ways. This "fix" creates a vicious cycle; as vision deteriorates, stronger prescriptions are needed. Corrective lenses address the symptoms of vision loss, doing nothing to solve the underlying problems.

By contrast, vision improvement techniques address the causes of vision problems. Losing your vision and wearing corrective lenses can often be avoided. You can learn eye exercises that prevent vision loss, and improving vision after it is impaired also is possible. Vision maintenance techniques enhance the strength and flexibility of the muscles and tissues of the eye, improving focus and clarity of vision at any distance:

- When reading or working at a computer, occasionally take a minute to look out the window at a distant object, studying the details of that object. This activity allows the eye muscles to relax. (Blankly gazing out the window does not make eye tissues return to their natural shape, whereas focusing on distant details does.) Do this once every thirty minutes or so for about a minute at a time. The exercise takes very little effort and helps to preserve your vision.

- If you wear corrective lenses, be sure to take them off whenever they are not needed, thus giving your eyes an opportunity to work naturally, especially when you are outdoors where the eyes can also receive full-spectrum light.

- For more tips on eyesight, see appendix E.

Reading, writing or sitting at a computer all day damages your eyesight, unless you take the time to rest and exercise your eyes—another important aspect of damage control on the physical pathway.

Heat Treatments Get Rid of Toxins

Not only do saunas feel good, they are good! Saunas get your heart beating and your blood circulating, helping the body to detoxify in unique and important ways. Toxins do the damage, and saunas help with damage control. Saunas or other heat treatments help to accomplish detoxification in the following manner: A layer of fat and oil exists just below the surface of the skin. Heat from the sauna increases skin temperature, causing those fats and oils to "melt" and ooze out of the skin's oil glands. As sweat and oil are secreted, the toxins dissolved in them are secreted as well. By excreting these toxins and then washing them off your body, your toxic load is lowered and cellular health improves.

Anything that raises the temperature of your skin for an extended period of time is helpful, including sweat wraps, steam rooms, hot baths and spas. Choose a temperature that can be tolerated for an extended period of time—thirty minutes to an hour or more. The point is not to sweat out a lot of water, but to rid your body of oil-soluble toxins. Our skin contains sweat glands and oil glands, both of which help us detoxify. Sweat gets rid of water-soluble toxins, and even helps to eliminate toxic heavy metals such as mercury and cadmium. Oil glands help remove oil-soluble toxins that the body would otherwise have a difficult time eliminating. We have created a world filled with oil-soluble toxins such as gasoline, solvents, pesticides and ingredients in toothpaste and personal care products, and the body is not able to dispose of them efficiently. The longer the skin is heated, the more oil-soluble toxins are eliminated.

Be careful not to overheat! The challenge is finding an environment where you can keep your skin temperature up for an extended period of time without overheating or dehydrating. Overheating and perhaps feeling dizzy can happen easily if you stay in a steam room, a hot tub or the top bench of a hot sauna too long. Choose a "low temperature" sauna (110–120 degrees), and use it for an extended period of time—an hour or more is best—though you may have to work up to this duration gradually. In a commercial sauna (which is usually too hot), try lying flat on the lowest bench. Remember: Drinking adequate amounts of water before, during and after your sauna is essential in order to prevent dehydration.

Every time I go to the gym to exercise, I spend an hour or more in the sauna, lying prone on the lowest bench to keep the temperature moderate. Sitting on the top bench in a high temperature for a short period of time does not aid in the elimination of oil-soluble toxins; effective elimination of these toxins takes time. A good supplement program, containing fat-mobilizing vitamins and essential fatty acids makes the sauna even more effective (see appendix B and C). Be sure to shower afterwards; prevent those toxins from reabsorbing back into your body by washing with a nontoxic Castile soap (see appendix C).

Taking saunas or other "heat treatments" is not a luxury, but like exercise, is a physical responsibility and an important element of the physical pathway. Incorporating saunas after exercise is even better. Exercise begins to mobilize toxins and saunas continue the process. You may need to make a few sauna visits before you can tolerate extended periods of time, but the benefits of these heat treatments are incredible. These treatments feel good for very good reasons; they provide beneficial physical stimulation—including increased lymphatic and cardiovascular circulation, as well as the removal of toxins—all of which are good for the health and function of your cells.

EMFs: Environmental Assault and Battery

Some forms of physical damage are obvious; others are invisible to the naked eye, such as electromagnetic radiation from sources such as medical X rays, microwaves, cell phones, TVs, power lines, broadcast antennae and other electrical items. Electromagnetic radiation can affect and damage our cells, leading to a variety of diseases including cancer.

The two kinds of electromagnetic radiation are ionizing and non-ionizing. Ionizing radiation (atom bombs, medical radiation, X rays) is the horrifying kind of radiation that we already know can injure and kill. Non-ionizing radiation (microwaves and electromagnetic fields) is easily overlooked and often labeled "benign." Non-ionizing radiation has measurable effects on cells and is therefore important to consider. Some scientists have made ominous statements about the effects on human health. The introduction of man-made electromagnetic pollution may indeed be the single most important environmental change we have made. Whenever possible, avoid exposing yourself to anything unnatural and foreign to the body, including all types of man-made electromagnetic energy.

Any electrical device—a hair dryer, TV set, electric blanket or dishwasher—produces a non-ionizing electromagnetic field (EMF) that affects the way our cells function. Cell membranes (or receptor molecules in them) act as amplifiers for sending signals into cells. EMFs can interrupt and change these signals, affecting certain cell functions and cell-to-cell communications. For example, EMFs can alter the rate at which cells make hormones, enzymes and other proteins. EMFs can also induce changes in the rate at which genetic material (DNA) is made and in the rate of errors when RNA is copied from it.

Researchers believe that daytime exposure to EMFs limits the release of melatonin, a cancer-protective and sleep-regulating hormone. By limiting release of melatonin, EMFs can contribute to cancer. One prominent cancer theory is that cancer cell growth results from a breakdown in cell-to-cell communication, which is precisely what happens when melatonin production is limited. In fact, any process that reduces the average level of melatonin is likely to promote estrogen-dependent cancers, such as breast, skin and prostate cancers.

Consider some examples of ominous EMF research: In 1998, a twenty-nine-member panel of the National Institute of Environmental Health Sciences concluded that there is a "possibility that electromagnetic fields are carcinogenic." The committee found a statistically significant correlation between EMF exposure and leukemia in both children and adults whose exposure was significantly higher than average. Likewise, studies in *Epidemiology* and the *American Journal of Epidemiology* have found statistically significant correlations between EMFs and breast cancer, brain cancer and Alzheimer's disease.

All of these health repercussions can occur simply from being near an electric appliance? Consider an experiment reported in scientist John Ott's 1976 book *Health and Light:* Two groups of mice were placed the same distance from a television set; one group was separated from the set by lead shielding, the other by black paper. The paper-shielded group became hyperactive, aggressive and wild, while the lead-shielded group remained normal. Autopsies of the paper-shielded group showed brain abnormalities. With studies like these, one wonders what may be happening to people who spend a lot of time in front of TV sets and computer monitors, particularly children whose brains are still developing and who are more sensitive to such damage. Is our children's behavior being affected not only by the messages on TV but also by radiation damage that we are not yet measuring? Less than a century ago, we did not sit in front of electronic screens at all; now we use them constantly, both at work and play.

The best policy for people concerned about health, especially cancer, is to minimize exposure to EMFs. Remember, EMFs are generated around electrical appliances, power lines and transformers; they can be found just about everywhere, including your home, office or school. EMFs become less dangerous as distance from the source increases, so choose to keep a safe distance between your body and electromagnetic fields.

How much exposure is too much? Scientists measure the power of these fields in miligauss (mG); experts around the world have proposed limiting chronic individual exposures to a level of 2 mG, with occasional peak exposures to about 10 mG. Unfortunately, we often experience much higher exposures. A hair dryer, which develops a powerful field next to your head, can dish out 20,000 mG. An electric razor (not a battery-powered razor) can generate 1,600 mG and is mere inches away from your pineal gland, which produces the cancer-protective hormone melatonin. A study done at Battel Memorial Institute's research center in Seattle found that men who used electric razors had twice the odds as nonusers of developing leukemia. The correlation between EMFs and cancer is positively alarming; we need to be careful!

A running dishwasher or clothes washer produces 30 to 50 mG at a distance of one foot, so be sure to keep a couple of feet away while it is running. A microwave oven can measure 80 mG at a distance of one foot, but quickly drops off to between 3 and 8 mG just thirty-nine inches away. A fluorescent lamp develops as much as 4,000 mG an inch away, but measures only 0.1 to 3 mG when thirty-nine inches away. A high voltage transmission line can measure up to 300 mG at the edge of the right-of-way; a regular distribution line can measure 80 mG right under the line. When buying a home or choosing an apartment, choose one that is not immediately adjacent to high-voltage distribution and transmission lines or transformers.

We need to be prudent in the use of appliances. When possible, use rechargeable battery-powered appliances rather than plug-in models. Do not stand immediately next to an electrical appliance when it is turned on, especially for an extended period of time. Follow these other recommendations also:

- Turn on the dishwasher when finished in the kitchen and you are ready to leave the room.

- Avoid electric blankets, or use them only to warm up the bed before you get in it.
- Keep telephone answering machines and electric clocks away from your head while you are sleeping.
- Increase distance from televisions (at least six feet away), computer monitors and appliances, especially those that come into close contact with your body, such as hair dryers and electric razors.
- Avoid using a cell phone. If you must use a cell phone, limit the number and length of your calls as much as possible.
- Avoid gazing into your microwave while your food warms up. Even better is to avoid the use of microwaves—for safety as well as nutritional and toxicological reasons—but at least stay a safe distance away if you do use one.
- Be careful of battery-powered wristwatches, a subtle but constant EMF exposure.
- Replace your computer monitor and television with flat panel display units, so as to eliminate the electromagnetic radiation emitted by the cathode ray tubes in regular TVs and monitors.

Of course, some people are more susceptible to EMFs than others (biochemical individuality at work). For example, people who are under stress seem to be more susceptible to damage by EMFs. In general, do whatever is possible to reduce EMF exposure—starting with the simple knowledge that these fields exist, realizing where they are and why they should be avoided.

Microwaves Zap More Than Food

Mobile phones produce a special kind of radiation called microwaves. Millions of us expose ourselves to a stream of microwaves every time we use our mobile phone for however long we talk. Cell phone microwaves are capable of damaging cellular DNA, thus contributing to cancer and other diseases. This damage can even be passed on to future generations. Research clearly shows that the microwaves produced by cell phones alter cell chemistry and function.

A Swedish study completed in 2001 by Professors Lennart Hardell and Kjell Hansson found that people who used cell phones for up to ten years had a 26 percent higher risk of brain cancer than a control sample who did not use cell phones. Mobile phone frequencies can cause a dramatic reduction in certain brain cell proteins and permanently damage brain cells; the cell phone antenna is right next to your brain.

Mast cells (cells involved with inflammatory responses such as those in asthma) were shown to be irreversibly damaged by exposure to mobile phone frequencies, with just ten minutes of exposure per day for seven days. Many people use their cell phones far more than that! To make matters worse, digital phones emit a series of pulses, and pulsed microwaves are known to be more biologically active than the continuous-wave radiation (analog phones) used in the experiments above. Cell phones can also interfere with melatonin production, thus interfering with sleep patterns and possibly promoting cancer. Since little research on the long-term effects of low-level microwave exposure has been done, the best course of action is to avoid cell phone use. When use is necessary, at least limit the number and duration of your calls.

The Threat of Ionizing Radiation

Ionizing radiation, as I have mentioned, is a serious kind of radiation that is fairly well known. This type of radiation, which includes gamma rays and X rays, is known to have harmful effects on human tissue. We call this type of radiation "ionizing" because it results in the formation of chemically reactive elements or molecules called ions, which alter the electrical charge in atoms and molecules within our cells. Ionizing radiation causes damage to DNA, cells, tissues and also causes cancer. Therefore, no level of exposure to radiation can be considered safe.

Research on ionizing radiation has uncovered many problems, from both natural and man-made sources. In 1983, residents of Montclair, New Jersey, began complaining of headaches and allergies. Their homes had been constructed on a landfill from a U.S. radium plant that closed in the 1930s. Their homes were found to be contaminated by "dangerously high" levels of radiation, which seemed to be related to the reported health problems. Similarly, in Kerela, India, which experiences the highest levels of natural environmental radiation in the world, a high prevalence of Down's syndrome and other forms of mental retardation are found among residents. Radiation damage is also evident in Japan's Hiroshima and Nagasaki victims and in the health records of former employees of government atomic facilities.

We have no control over about half of the ionizing radiation we are exposed to in our lives, because it comes from natural sources such as radioactive elements in our soil, water and atmosphere. Research the level of radiation in the ground and water where you live. If your local ambient radiation is particularly high, you might want to consider a different home. At least avoid drinking contaminated water and use ventilation to remove radioactive gas from your basement.

We do have control over the other half of the ionizing radiation we are exposed to—that which comes from man-made sources, primarily medical X rays. Seemingly "benign" dental X rays, mammograms and other radiological procedures can subject the body to significant physical harm. Given that the overwhelming majority of diagnostic X rays are not medically necessary, we should consider them as a health risk and carefully evaluate their value (risks versus benefits). Whether or not to have an X ray is your choice, not your doctor's, and the decision should be made by you. As noted, this decision should not be taken lightly because ionizing radiation from medical X rays and radiation treatment can cause cancer, genetic defects and tissue injury.

In the medical and scientific communities, much disagreement exists about the health effects of low-level exposure to ionizing radiation in diagnostic procedures. Many have assumed that low-level exposure is not a health threat, but modern research is beginning to cast doubts. A study of the health records of thirty-five thousand workers at a government bomb plant in Washington state concluded that even small doses of ionizing radiation are four to eight times more likely to cause cancer than previously believed. This study, financed by the Three Mile Island Public Health Fund and carried out by Alice Stewart, M.D., concluded that *radiation delivered in small doses over time (as we are exposed to today through common medical X rays) may carry a higher risk of cancer than the same total radiation delivered in a single dose.*

Edward Radford, past chairman of the National Academy of Sciences committee on ionizing radiation, says the cancer risk of low-level radiation may be ten times worse than is generally accepted. Higher radiation doses may kill off damaged cells, thus preventing their proliferation, whereas weak exposures damage cellular DNA but still allow damaged cells to replicate; thus, cells are able to reproduce and proliferate cancerous mutations. This conclusion is the opposite of what our dentists and physicians teach us; the medical community has always maintained that X rays are safe because small doses over time give the body time to repair itself and are therefore less damaging. However, instead of repairing, the body's cells appear to suffer damage and then replicate that damage, enabling the problem to spread.

The bottom line: Avoid radiation whenever possible. Because some radiation exists in the natural world, we must focus on reducing our exposure to the radiation we create, especially from medical X rays.

Optimizing Your Physical Pathway

This chapter began with a comparison between your body and your car. Your car will provide better service and last longer if you take good care of it. Even an old, beat-up car can be restored to good function with tender loving care. The same is true of your body. To move yourself in the right direction on the physical pathway, maintain your body—with good nutrition, exercise, sleep, proper breathing and natural sunlight—and protect your body from physical harm, including loud noises, sunburn and radiation. Making even minor adjustments to your physical pathway can make a big difference. As always, the choice is yours.

9

THE GENETIC PATHWAY

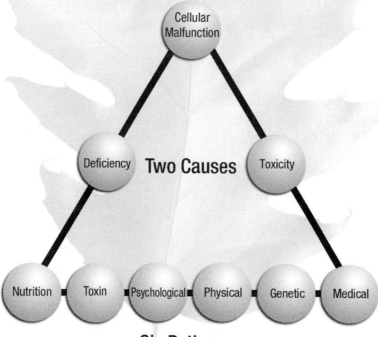

"Genetics may load the gun, but environment pulls the trigger."

Pamela Peeke, M.D., M.P.H.
Fight Fat After Forty

One of the most manipulated terms in conversations about health is the word "genetic." Almost weekly in the news, genetic discoveries are announced, proclaiming the genetic origins of a myriad of problems—from cancer to compulsive shopping. Scientists usually describe a gene as being associated with a particular disease (rather than directly causing it), but the details become distorted and misinterpreted. Many are confused about what genes are and how they work. *We end up being misled into believing that genes control health directly—which is not accurate, because the environment we create for our cells controls the expression of our genes.*

While true genetic diseases do exist, they affect less than 5 percent of the population. Heredity is trumped by environment, and you control your environment. You have control over the rate at which you age and the diseases that you will (or will not) develop. Turn the right genes on, and keep the wrong genes off. Health is not about genes; it is about cells. Once again, we are in charge. Use the six pathways to optimize the health of your cells, and you control the expression of your genes.

Will the Weakest Link Fail?

What about the genetic predisposition to disease we hear so much about? What about health problems that "run in the family"?

Think of a genetic predisposition to disease as a weak link in a chain—a weak link with the potential to break, but only if excessively stressed. In the right environment, the weak link will function just fine. If the chain does break (if sickness does occur), it is not accurate to say that the weak link (the "bad" gene) is the sole trigger of the problem. Excess biological stress is the trigger, and this we can control.

By enhancing the function of cells, genetic predispositions can remain potential problems, rather than becoming real problems, regardless of what "runs in the family." Unfortunately, people often give up to their genetic predispositions, relieving themselves—at least in their own minds—of responsibility for their actions. The genetically predisposed person might say nonchalantly, "There is nothing I can do; weight problems run in my family" (as they gulp down a burger, fries and large shake). The thinking that genes and germs are the primary factors determining our state of health is outdated and fatalistic. Genes and germs are factors worth considering, but they are not the causes of disease that we typically understand them to be.

Let us consider genes, what they are, how they work, and what we all can do to put the potential for health back into our own hands, regardless of which genes we have inherited.

Nature Versus Nurture

Genes are the blueprints or "plans" for life; they are the instructions that tell our bodies how to develop from one single cell into an entire human being. However, only about one-quarter of our genes express ("turn on") automatically, determining, for example, whether our eyes are blue or our hair is curly. Imagine most other genes as a set of coded instructions that, much like a computer program, sit dormant, essentially doing nothing, until you activate them.

Most genes require some sort of trigger (environmental or psychological) in order for them to express. Just because a certain trait, "bad" or "good," runs in the family does not mean that every person in the family possesses that trait or will express it even if they possess it. We often worry far more than we need to about genetic inheritance. *Most important is the environment you create for your cells based on what you eat and how you live your life.* You cannot control your heredity; you can control the environment you create for your cells.

Rather than thinking of genes as an absolute and unchanging set of instructions, one might think of them as a variety of possibilities—a set of "what if" instructions. If certain circumstances are present, then a person's genes express in a particular way; if other circumstances are present, those same genes express in a different way. Biochemist Roger Williams maintained that genes alone are entirely useless threads of chemicals. Genes alone do not determine our sickness or health.

If genes, in the form of cellular DNA, were the primary control of the cell—if they were the "brain" of a cell, so to speak—then the cell would die without them, but this does not happen. Scientists commonly perform a process called denucleation, a process whereby the nucleus of a cell and its DNA are removed. After this process, cells continue to perform normal functions for months.

Consider how changes in diet, lifestyle and environment over the past one hundred years have coincided with massive increases in rates of chronic disease. For example, in 1900 cancer affected only 3 percent of the U.S. population; now about 50 percent of all men and 40 percent of all women develop cancer in their lifetime. Our environment has changed so radically that blaming disease increases solely on inherited genes is illogical.

Consider how environmental factors can affect genetic expression. Environmental temperature, for example, affects the expression of genes that control the coloration of Himalayan rabbits. These rabbits, accustomed to cold temperatures, usually have black ears, forepaws, noses and tails, but when raised in warm temperatures they have no black markings at all. Same rabbits, same genes, but different environments and, therefore, different expressions of genes. Similarly, plants with the genetic capacity to flower and fruit only do so when a precise set of environmental requirements (such as temperature, sunlight and moisture) "turn on" the necessary genes. "Disease genes" function the same way. When people move from one part of the world to another—adopting the diet and lifestyle habits of the new environment—they also develop the disease conditions common to that new environment. For example, people from countries with low rates of heart disease and cancer, such as Japan, suffer like the rest of our population once they move here.

A compelling question in the discussion of heredity is how long you will live—your life span. A low-calorie diet is the only thing that consistently has been shown to increase life span. Genetic expression causes this to happen. A study in the September 2001 *Proceedings of the National Academy of Sciences* found that a high-calorie diet (the typical American diet) caused changes in genes that reduced the expression of disease-protective genes and turned on genes that accelerate the aging process. But the good news is that the study also showed that by taking older animals and putting them on calorie-restricted diets for merely four weeks, about half of the gene expressions that were contributing to the aging process reversed. *Changing internal cellular environment (by reducing calories) not only helps to prevent the expression of aging genes in the young, it can also slow and even reverse the aging process in the old.*

As biologist Steven Rose pointed out in his 1997 book, *Lifelines,* much of what goes on in a cell is at least as much a product of the environment in and around the cell as its DNA. This environment is something we create with our diet, toxic exposures, lifestyle, and even with our thoughts, beliefs and perceptions. "Organisms," Rose wrote, "are active players in their own fate."

Indeed, even mental climate affects the environment we create for our cells and genes. Cells depend on the brain to interpret the environment and to use the nervous system to relay that information, telling the cells what to do. Depending on one's perceptions of the environment, the expression of genes can be greatly affected. For example, the mortality rate goes up during the first year or two after retirement. Why? Does the brain perceive that "life" is over, causing the genes to express accordingly? Deepak Chopra, M.D., author of many books and a pioneer and leader in mind/body medicine, often says in his lectures, "Aging is a mistake." He means that we observe others around us aging, so we believe that we too will age. We literally instruct our genes to age us. Could this be one of the reasons that traditionally healthy people like the Hunzas lived so long? By believing that they would live long, healthy lives, did they actually instruct their genes accordingly? Much evidence indicates that what we believe does affect the function of our cells and the expression of our genes.

Intentional Damage to Your DNA

Modern diet and lifestyle can cause damage to genes—different from genetically inherited predispositions. Rather than causing the expression of existing genetic coding, genetic damage involves changes in the coding. A change in genetic coding is known as a mutation, which can occur both through natural causes and man-created damage. One theory of aging is that gene mutations over a lifetime cause gradual loss of function and resilience. The ability of genes to mutate is not all "bad," but rather is an essential part of evolution and of adaptation to changing conditions.

The mutations to be concerned about are caused by chemicals and radiation, which can lead to dramatic and unpredictable changes in genetic coding. Genes are crucial plans for creating, repairing and reproducing an organism; randomly changing these plans is a bad idea. What would happen if you started making random changes to the blueprints of your house? Doors, windows, walls and even whole rooms would appear in strange places. So it is with genetic damage.

What causes genetic mutation?

- *Ionizing radiation:* Almost half of the average person's exposure to ionizing radiation comes from medical X rays and medical radiation treatments. Avoid this kind of radiation unless vitally necessary. It's bizarre that physicians put much stock in the genetic origins of disease yet also inflict massive amounts of genetic damage with pharmaceutical chemicals and X rays.
- *Non-ionizing radiation:* This is created by the flow of electricity and may also have genetic repercussions—though the evidence is less clear. As a general rule, avoid close proximity or prolonged exposure to all types of electric devices.
- *Toxins:* These include man-made industrial chemicals, prescription drugs, tobacco, alcohol and chemical

residues in meat and dairy products, such as PCBs and dioxins. In particular, foods that are heated to high temperatures or blackened (such as in barbecuing) contain chemicals capable of causing gene mutations and cancer.

When a cell is exposed to toxins or radiation, the cell may die or the genes may be damaged. A mutated gene may permanently alter the way the cell works, often contributing to deficiency, toxicity and disease. Furthermore, altered cells (with mutated genes) can replicate, allowing the mutation to propagate throughout more and more cells. The effects of this replication can range from minor to devastating; replication is a classic way for cancer to develop. Worse, if genetic mutations take place in a reproductive cell, a 50/50 chance exists of passing these on to an unborn child. Destroyed or damaged cells and genes can lead to premature aging and a variety of diseases, including cancer, fatigue, poor resistance to infections, psychological stress and even social maladjustment.

Genes are not causing aging and disease. We are. We expose our cells to the toxins and radiation that make the genes mutate in the first place. Life in the twenty-first century is now causing damage to our genes and creating mutations in unprecedented ways and at an alarming rate. As scientist Richard Lewontin said in his 1982 book, *Human Diversity:* "Because of technology's ventures into ionizing radiation and synthetic chemistry, the human beings of our age, as well as the food chain on which we live, are thought to be undergoing a far higher mutation rate than biology has been accustomed to."

Fortunately, under the right circumstances, genetic damage can be repaired. Not only must we avoid damaging our genes in the first place, we also must provide our genes with the materials (nutrients) they need in order to repair themselves.

Genetically Modified Foods: Risky Business

No contemporary discussion on genetics is complete without discussing the powerful genetic technologies in use today, particularly with our foods. With modern genetic technology, what would have seemed miraculous just a generation ago is now possible. However, whether or not these technologies pose a threat to our health is a huge debate. Scientists on both sides constantly argue their points. These technologies present the potential both for great achievement and for catastrophe. Not enough research is available to know what will happen, although the research that is available presents cause for serious concern or even alarm. I recommend against consuming genetically modified foods because I believe these foods may be lower in nutrients, higher in toxins and present other potential risks as well.

Never before in human evolution has humankind eaten a genetically modified food. Only in recent years have we developed the technologies that allow us to create these foods. Now genetic technologies are being developed and deployed rapidly, with few controls and almost no consideration for long-term consequences. Most of the food in your supermarket already contains genetically modified components. Yet there is insufficient research, particularly long-term research, to establish the safety of genetically modified foods and, indeed, ample reason to believe they may not be safe.

If we keep producing and consuming genetically modified foods, we will be unable to prevent genetic contamination from becoming prevalent throughout our entire food supply. If ever these foods are determined unsafe, the damage will be irreversible. Unexpected results from these foods might not become obvious until years after they are introduced, at which point taking it back is too late. Our scientists do their best, but when experimenting with genetics, the potential for unanticipated side effects is almost incalculable. Here is one scenario: Over time, genetically modified organisms interact with their environment, mutate and evolve, and pass on their mutant characteristics to other related and unrelated organisms, including us. This sets off a chain of events throughout the entire ecosystem, jeopardizing life on earth as we know it. I know this scenario sounds dramatic, but messing with genes and the course of evolution is risky business.

Is That a Jellyfish in Your Potato?

Producing new foods with modern genetic engineering is no minor event. Genetic engineers cut, splice and transfer genes between totally unrelated species to produce combinations that could never occur in nature. Scientists are inserting jellyfish genes into potatoes, scorpion genes into vegetables, human genes into pigs and fish genes into tomatoes. Perfect accuracy using these gene-splicing techniques and knowing exactly what will be produced is almost impossible. Researchers at the prestigious Rowett Institute in Scotland studied different batches of genetically modified potatoes and found substantial differences from the same gene insertion. Two lines of potatoes grown from the same gene insertion and the same growing conditions had a 20 percent difference in protein content, demonstrating the unpredictability inherent in genetic modification.

Genetically modified foods may be of altered nutritional value, and they also may contain allergens or toxins they would not naturally contain—including ones not normally associated with that type of food. For example, genes from Brazil nuts were used to engineer a new soybean; but people allergic to Brazil nuts were now highly reactive to these soybeans. Fortunately the problem was discovered before anyone was harmed. Other genetically modified foods may present similar risks. A 1999 study printed in the British medical journal *Lancet* showed that genetically modified potatoes damaged the stomach and intestinal linings of rats. People are also eating genetically modified potatoes, but similar tests are not being performed on humans.

Do you recall one of the health "scandals" of the late 1980s? Many people who took an essential amino acid called tryptophan (which is used for treating depression and other emotional problems) had devastating reactions. Thirty-seven people died, fifteen hundred were permanently disabled, and five thousand became extremely ill. As it turned out, one particular manufacturer in Japan had produced tryptophan using a genetically modified bacterium, which did produce commercial quantities of tryptophan, but which also produced a powerful nerve poison. Of course this poison did not exist until we created it with genetic engineering, so it could not be detected by existing safety tests. We cannot test for toxins we don't know about, which is the problem with genetically engineered foods. They are capable of producing the unexpected.

Supermarkets Full of Genetic Experiments

Food industry journals estimate that about 70 percent of the processed foods in our supermarkets would test positive for genetically modified ingredients. Most common are genetically engineered corn, soybeans, tomatoes, yellow crookneck squash, canola, papaya and Russet Burbank potatoes. Other foods are being developed, such as apples, rice, wheat, broccoli, cucumbers, carrots, melons and grapes; genetically modified versions of these foods are either in stores already or they soon will be.

A 1999 study by *Consumer Reports* found that only one-third of U.S. shoppers realize they are eating genetically modified foods. The FDA does not require these foods to be labeled "genetically modified," and consumers do not realize what they are buying. People buy so-called "fresh" produce, unaware that these foods did not evolve through a natural process. As always, your best bet is to purchase only fresh, organic foods. If you are unable to buy organic, stay away from commercial foods most likely to be genetically modified, particularly corn and soy (including tofu). Avoid commercially processed and prepared foods, 70 percent of which contain genetically modified components, often including soy as a hidden ingredient.

Even organic foods are not guaranteed to be free from genetically modified components. Segregating organic crops completely from genetically modified crops during harvest, handling, transport and milling is not possible. Similarly, insects, birds and wind carry seeds and pollen from genetically modified plants into organic fields and cross-pollinate. America's crops are so contaminated by genetic modification that the Organic Federation of Australia announced in 2001 that it could no longer verify the purity of organic crops imported from the United States. Closer to home, Farm Verified Organic, an organic certification agency, has stated, "the GM [genetically modified] pollution of American commodities is now so pervasive, we believe it is not possible for farmers in North America to source seed free from it." Our supposedly uncontaminated organic crops of corn, soy and canola are now testing positive for the presence of foreign genetic material.

As you know, commercial farming produces sick plants, which are sprayed with chemical fertilizers and pesticides to keep them alive. To cut down on pesticide use, some genetically modified crops (such as corn and potatoes) have been engineered to produce toxic pesticides internally. These plants actually become their own pesticide factories. The long-term health effects of these pesticides are unknown. With such crops, the potential certainly exists for long-term nutritional deficiencies, toxicities and even genetic mutations in humans. A December 1999 issue of *Nature* reported that genetically modified crops engineered to produce their own pesticides actually were poisoning the soil. Pesticides leaching from the plant's roots were killing beneficial bacteria in the soil, disrupting the soil food web and threatening soil ecology. This problem is severe. The quality of the soil has everything to do with the health and nutritional content of the crops it produces.

Genetically modified organisms are problematic because they are extremely hard to control. Genes do not exist by themselves. They exist as part of interactive networks. The splicing of genes results in not only the desired characteristics but also in other unpredictable effects. Given that the species developed by Mother Nature work just fine, why take these unnecessary risks?

"Progress?" At What Price?

The companies that supply genetically modified seeds, such as Archer Daniels Midland and Monsanto, believe they are pioneers in a technology that can serve humankind and offer myriad benefits now and in the future. Scientists in this field argue that genetically modified foods increase yields and are necessary to feed this hungry world. They argue that crops can be engineered to reduce environmental pesticide pollution, because pesticides are produced internally by the plants. They argue that the plants can be engineered to resist chemical weed killers, so farmers can use these chemicals without fear of harming crops. Future possibilities include engineering plants that are better able to withstand harsh environmental conditions, permitting farming in areas not presently suitable. Another possibility is the engineering of crops with increased nutritional content. Clearly, genetically modified foods present great promise, but as always, we must consider the whole picture.

These foods also present enormous risks for which there is little financial incentive to investigate and plenty of incentive to overlook. Safety tests for these newly created species should be at least as rigorous as those for new food additives, but they are not. No single regulatory agency is in charge of genetically modified foods. Eight government agencies are involved under twelve different laws, none of which deal specifically with genetically modified foods. Biotechnology companies do their own testing and are not required to inform the FDA if they suspect a problem. Huge corporations and large sums of money are involved, yet we rely on the honor system alone. At the very least, people have a right to know what they are eating. We should insist that genetically engineered foods be labeled as such. In order to make our voices heard, contact your elected representatives and tell them what you think.

Misleading Thoughts About Birth Defects

One of the central points of confusion regarding genetics and disease is the common misunderstanding between genetic and congenital defects. Most people assume that a condition present at birth is genetically determined. Not so. In a newborn baby, the environmental conditions in the womb contributed to every step of its development. Defects caused by problematic conditions in the womb are congenital, not genetic.

Building a baby puts a huge demand on the mother, which can be met only with a much higher than normal intake of nutrients. Grave consequences often affect the developing fetus if a mother fails to obtain proper nutrition. *Congenital defects—biochemical and physical defects present at birth— are not determined by genes, but by the same two causes responsible for all disease: deficiency and toxicity.*

If the mother's cells are neither deficient nor toxic, her baby's chances for a healthy life increase dramatically. As a fetus passes through various developmental stages, tissues and cells grow very quickly. Rapidly dividing cells are at a greater risk of suffering from insufficient nutrients, too much of certain hormones or the presence of certain toxins. These conditions can alter the development of the baby's tissues, permanently affecting the physical and mental function of the child.

An unfavorable environment in the womb causes a developing fetus to make compromises in order to compensate for deficiency or toxicity. These compensations come at a very high price, a price that often is invisible and impossible to measure. Perhaps the newborn's nervous system is compromised and the child's IQ will be lower than it might otherwise be. Perhaps the baby's digestive system is not fully developed, leading to digestive problems, disease and shortened life span. Perhaps the circulatory system is not fully developed, making it impossible for optimal amounts of nutrients and oxygen to reach the tissues, thus guaranteeing premature aging and disease. Perhaps the baby is born with a cleft palate, a clubfoot or a heart defect.

Some of these problems are obvious at birth, but most are not. When they are obvious, we usually blame them on genetics, but they are mostly congenital. To avoid these problems, parents, especially prior to and during pregnancy, must follow the six pathways closely, optimizing their cellular function and minimizing the chances of congenital problems in their children.

Choosing Your Destiny

Although perfect nutrition, perfect genes, a pure environment and ideal behavior do not exist, these factors write the story of your life, including how many chapters you will finish. *The interaction between inherited genes, nutritional intake, the environment and our beliefs at any point in time are the triggers that determine our current state of health or disease, including how long we live.*

By changing the conditions inside your body, you can signal your genes to express in different ways. Our society tends to think that disease is the result of aging. Not true. The Hunzas and other historically healthy populations lived to very old ages without disease. Disease is a result of the rate at which we age, not the number of years we have inhabited the Earth. The rate is affected by "aging genes," which we can choose to keep turned off.

You can create a younger and healthier you, as was suggested by Arthur Vander, M.D., in his 1981 book, *Nutrition, Stress, & Toxic Chemicals: An Approach to Environmental-Health Controversies.* Dr. Vander said, "Different environments, by altering gene expression, can produce . . . an incredible variety of 'yous.'"

By assuming that inherited genes cause disease, one assumes that disease occurs regardless of dietary and lifestyle factors—in other words, environment. Not so, which is why we can have such a powerful influence on the balance between health and disease. Genes are important, but they are only one small piece of a much larger puzzle. Fundamentally, there is only one disease (malfunctioning cells), and it has only two causes (deficiency and toxicity).

Regardless of the recipe you start with, a dish is only as good as the ingredients put into it. The same goes for a cell. When a cell is provided with the proper nutrients, kept free from toxins and placed in a supportive environment, health-supporting genes are activated, aging and disease-causing genes remain dormant, and both your cells and you are healthy. To move yourself in the right direction on the genetic pathway, create a healthy environment for your genes and protect them from damage.

10

THE MEDICAL PATHWAY

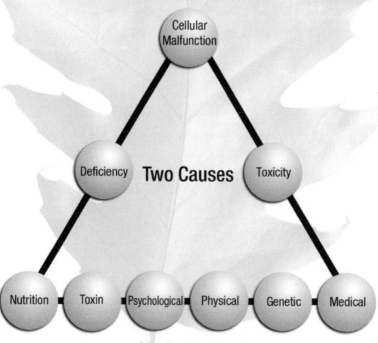

One Disease

Cellular Malfunction

Deficiency **Two Causes** Toxicity

Nutrition   Toxin   Psychological   Physical   Genetic   Medical

Six Pathways

"[T]he greatest danger to your health is the doctor who practices Modern Medicine."

Robert Mendelsohn, M.D.
Confessions of a Medical Heretic

One spring morning, more than twenty years ago, I received a call from my father's physician telling me that my father, hospitalized for emphysema, was dying of kidney failure. I raced to the hospital almost two hundred miles away. My brother and I found our father in a deep coma. He looked as if he were dead.

The doctors advised us to disconnect his life-support systems and allow him to slip away peacefully. We knew our father would not choose to live hooked to machines in a vegetative state. We knew his own decision would be to pull the plug. We consented. All life-support measures were terminated.

Late that evening, our father was still alive but in a deep coma. In the morning, my brother and I returned to the hospital with anxiety and grief. We thought that he might have died during the night. Instead, we found our father sitting up and telling jokes to the nurse!

A miracle? No. The doctors had been giving our father

"life-saving" prescription drugs that put a lethal load of toxins on his kidneys. When the drugs were stopped, his body was able to rebalance and begin to repair itself. A night without the drugs was sufficient. Our decision to "let him die" saved him. Had he died, his death would have been attributed to kidney failure, not the prescription drugs that were causing his kidneys to fail.

My father's story is extreme, yet all too common. The vast number of medically caused deaths is underreported and underestimated. Prescription errors, surgical mistakes and missed diagnoses do not even begin to describe the scope of the problem. The truth is lost in prescription pads, health charts and death certificates, which do not reflect the true causes of death and disease. We pride ourselves on the accomplishments of modern medicine without acknowledging its failures. Actually, *medical intervention may be the leading cause of death in the United States.*

Conventional medical treatments can be both a blessing or a curse. These treatments are good, even excellent, in crisis intervention and treatment of injuries. But conventional medicine does not prevent nor cure disease; it manages symptoms. We wait for disease to happen, wait for the damage to be done and then try to control the problems by "treating," using assembly-line techniques that are currently fashionable, expensive and usually dangerous. These techniques cause cellular malfunction—often cavalierly called "side effects"—which lead to unnecessary suffering, disease and death. Even so-called preventive medicine usually is only early disease detection, rather than real prevention.

The present system suffers from a disease-care bias. Very few medical resources are devoted to disease prevention by helping people to maintain cellular health through diet, nutritional supplements, detoxification, exercise, healthful environment, state of mind and lifestyle. Instead, resources are devoted toward treating the effects of disease. Our modern medical system fails to find cures for chronic diseases despite vast sums of money spent on research every year. The late Emanuel Cheraskin, M.D., D.M.D., at the University of Alabama Medical Center, said, "American medical care is the fastest-growing failing business in Western Civilization."

The Truth and the Consequences

Many people maintain total and unquestioning trust in modern medicine. They get advice and treatments from only one school of thought and willingly surrender their personal health responsibilities to the hands of their doctor. This approach is not sensible. *Educate yourself before you follow anyone else's advice, including your physician's.* Health is the responsibility of the individual.

Rarely do most people realize that certain aspects of medicine might harm their health, or that better alternatives might exist. Instead, they do what is familiar and conventional. Confronted with a health problem, they go to the doctor either because they do not know how to solve the problem or they are intimidated by alternatives. This was certainly my experience.

The medical pathway teaches you how all kinds of medical treatments affect your body at the cellular level, the benefits and the dangers. With this understanding, and if you are not blinded by unquestioning trust in modern medicine, you can evaluate the evidence and make the best choices about medical care for yourself and for your family. With the right health choices, you should not become sick. But if you do, you must take an active part in your care which means more than blindly following someone else's advice. You need to learn how to take charge—relying on medicine alone is not a sensible long-term solution.

Like most people in our society, I grew up wholeheartedly trusting modern medicine. When I became sick I took my physicians' advice without question and believed that I was benefiting from the most advanced medical science and the most effective treatments. I unwittingly waited in line at the pharmacy for my toxic drugs. Not until I almost died as a direct result of my medical treatments did I question the validity of this approach, and then it was almost too late. Before choosing any medical treatment, consider both benefits and risks. Understand your choices and how they are supposed to benefit you, and find out the risks.

What Is Not on the Death Certificate

A physician may actually guide your movement along the pathways toward disease rather than away from it. That happened to Harry, a delightful seventy-two-year-old man and a dear friend. I was shocked to hear that Harry had died of pneumonia. His story is important to relate.

Although Harry's pneumonia was caused by a bacterial infection, healthy people rarely develop infections, especially serious ones. Generally, infections occur in people who are already unhealthy, whose cells are malfunctioning and whose immunity is already compromised. Harry had always been a strong, healthy person who rarely succumbed to colds or flu. That pneumonia caused his death seemed suspicious. Something must have happened to make him susceptible to the infection that killed him. I sadly surmised that, most likely, modern medicine killed Harry.

Harry had been suffering pain in his hip from a congenital problem. His doctor prescribed a steroid hormone, cortisone. This drug helps alleviate pain and inflammation, but it has nasty side effects. Cortisone damages the immune system by inhibiting the production of antibodies and "killer" T-cells. In addition, this damage makes localizing infections difficult if they develop. The cortisone made Harry vulnerable to infection. He developed pneumonia in one lung and was hospitalized, where he was given large doses of antibiotics—presumably to kill the "germs" causing the pneumonia. Pneumonia, like any infection, is caused by malfunctioning cells and depressed immunity, not by germs alone. Normalizing cell function and rebuilding immunity, rather than trying to kill germs, is needed for recovery. But that is not what happened in Harry's case: After a few days on antibiotics, he was discharged, supposedly "cured."

In reality, the antibiotics had increased Harry's problems because they further compromised his immunity. His already depressed immune system was now in worse shape than before. Shortly after returning home Harry developed another infection. This time the pneumonia affected both lungs, and shortly thereafter he died. During his first hospitalization, Harry became infected with a "superbug," an antibiotic-resistant germ that is now common in hospitals. Antibiotics were useless against this infection, as was Harry's damaged immune system. In all likelihood, the state-of-the-art medical establishment both destroyed Harry's immune system and subjected him to the untreatable infection that killed him. Yet, the death certificate stated the official cause of death as pneumonia.

At my sickest, I was dying from liver failure that resulted from the toxic effects of a prescription drug. If I had died, guess what cause would have been listed on my death certificate? Liver disease. Period. No mention of the drug that made me sick would have been recorded.

Only in the most blatant and obvious cases does modern medicine consider or take responsibility for the damage it causes. Fears of malpractice claims only enhance the resolve of the medical community to keep listing causes of death as resulting from the sickness of the patient, rather than the treatments of the doctor. Physicians usually assume that the health problems they cause would have happened anyway. The general belief is that the negative effects of drugs and procedures are worth the risk. Little wonder that the cause of death on death certificates often has to do with the specialty of the doctor treating the disease.

Prescriptions for Trouble

To understand the extent of the damage caused by the medical establishment, consider how the patient can be sent toward disease along the six pathways:

- Medical treatments can cause nutritional deficiencies. Antibiotics, anti-inflammatories and steroid prescription drugs seriously damage the human digestive system, impairing the ability to digest food and absorb nutrients. Diuretics strip nutrients such as magnesium, calcium, potassium, zinc and iodine.
- Drugs work because they are toxic; they interfere with normal cell function, in order to suppress disease symptoms. Both prescription and over-the-counter drugs produce a vast variety of disease symptoms referred to as *side effects.*
- Often physicians inflict psychological damage on their patients. When doctors estimate how long a patient will live, or predict that the patient will never walk or see again, they can create a self-fulfilling prophecy. Often physicians don't even listen to their patients' thoughts and opinions, interrupting them less than a minute after the patients start describing symptoms. Such practices sabotage one of the physician's primary goals: to help and support the patient throughout the entire healing process.
- Many medical procedures, including surgery, medical X rays and radiation, physically damage the body and ultimately cause malfunction and disease. This physical damage can lead to genetic damage. Genetic mutations can cause cancer and other diseases, and may be passed to future generations.

Managing Symptoms
Instead of Curing Disease

If you seek medical treatment, your physician asks you a series of questions and, perhaps, runs a series of tests to determine your symptoms. The purpose of this activity is to diagnose—to match your set of symptoms with specific named categories, also known as diseases. Diagnosed in this manner, a disease is nothing more than a set of symptoms. After diagnosis, modern medicine (also known as "allopathic" medicine; "allo" = against, and "pathic" = disease) literally seeks to "go against" the symptoms of disease.

Symptoms are significant only because they attract your attention; they are unpleasant and interfere with your ability to function, but they have nothing to do with the essence of health and disease. Disease ensues when cells malfunction. The symptoms may vary, the solution is always the same: Normalize cell function through the six pathways.

Perception is everything. Perceived symptoms become the "problem" that medicine seeks to stop. For example, if the perceived problem is high blood pressure, medicine aims to lower pressure with a variety of toxic drugs. If the perceived problem is a germ, medicine aims to kill the germ with toxic antibiotics. Meanwhile, both of these problems are merely symptoms of malfunctioning cells. Using drugs to lower the blood pressure, therefore, does not solve the problem that is causing the elevated pressure. And likewise with drugs used to kill germs. Germs can contribute to cellular malfunction, but germs are present constantly and everywhere in our environment. Killing the germs that are causing an infection does not make the person healthy, nor does it make the person more resistant to subsequent infections. In fact, they become less resistant because the drugs that kill the germs also damage and weaken the body.

When one has an infection, masking the symptoms of the

sickness (fever, etc.) serves little purpose other than making
the sick person more comfortable. For example, treating fever
with over-the-counter drugs is a common practice. Yet, fever
is natural and beneficial; there is no reason to use drugs for
this purpose, especially because the drugs inflict harm.

By focusing on symptoms and taking drugs, we do not cure
disease; we merely invent ways to allow sick people to continue living their lives more comfortably. Short-term relief has
its place but is not a long-term solution. For example, angio-
plasty may prevent the immediate death of a patient by
increasing blood flow to the heart; however, only by eliminating deficiency and toxicity can the heart disease be reversed,
and this will not happen under the guidance of a conventional
physician.

More Than a Sum of Our Parts

Modern medicine, pumped up with huge amounts of talent
and money, is a strange dichotomy—technologically
advanced and cutting-edge, yet obsolete and ineffective.
Medicine does a superb job managing medical emergencies
and disease symptoms, but is woefully incapable of curing
disease or promoting a lifetime of wellness. In medical
schools, physicians study one organ or system at a time and
then specialize, without developing an understanding of health
or the body as a whole. A lack of holistic understanding and
appreciation transfers to medicine's focus on disease rather
than health.

Actually, our modern health-care system is a disease-care
system. Our health-care providers are paid for treating disease, not for preventing disease. Treatments can continue for
the entire life of the patient. Our current system does not offer
financial incentives for health, but provides a lot of money for
treatments of disease.

We need to examine the roots of modern conventional

medicine. "Modern medicine" is based on a seventeenth-century understanding of the human body, and it has failed to incorporate the most important scientific discoveries of the twentieth century. Wrapped in the cloak of modern science, at its core, *conventional medicine is based on archaic concepts that presently are scientifically obsolete and invalid.* Allow me to explain what I mean.

Beginning with Isaac Newton's discovery of the laws of motion, the human body and the universe both became regarded as a clockwork mechanism. From this perspective, anything can be dissected into parts, studied scientifically and understood. Medicine of the time followed this mechanistic concept: Take the machine apart, study the parts, understand how they work and use that understanding in medical care. People began to believe they could control health simply by understanding the mechanical workings of the physical body. Many people still believe this, although it isn't true. Today the medical establishment continues to regard the body as a complex, glorified machine; the focus is on the parts, not the whole.

Disease is seen as confined to specific locations or organs, rather than as affecting the whole person. Treatments regularly remove or replace body parts without addressing the reasons that something went awry. By assuming the body is a machine that cannot heal itself, the only effective therapies are thought to be those that come from the outside, such as mechanical techniques, surgical invasion and powerful drugs. The pharmaceutical drug industry "fixes" health problems by adding molecules to the body that are designed to control the function of certain body parts, without seeking to understand or remedy the reasons for the malfunction. A dysfunction in the body's self-regulating and balancing mechanisms is caused by cellular malfunction, and it affects the whole body, not just a part of it. With machines, the function of the whole can be predicted by the sum of the parts, but humans are not machines. A living organism is much greater than the sum of its parts. We are alive, and our minds influence our bodies.

In the early twentieth century, Albert Einstein challenged existing perceptions and fundamentally changed the way people view the world. By proving that matter and energy are one, Einstein brought forth a new field for studying the laws of the universe, quantum physics, in which human beings are regarded as networks of complex energy systems that interact with physical and cellular systems.

We human beings are not Newtonian in nature, but rather Einsteinian. Humans are matter, but we are also multidimensional energy systems, and our thoughts, beliefs and attitudes create energy fields that influence our biochemistry and affect our health. Yet our physicians continue to use the mechanical Newtonian model.

No Ground to Stand On

We are brought up to think of medicine as scientific and that the techniques and procedures used by our physicians are the result of extensive scientific study. Not so. Several studies, including a 1978 report by the U.S. Office of Technology Assessment, have estimated that no scientific basis exists for 80 to 90 percent of all procedures used in medical practice.

In fact, traditional or allopathic medicine has no general theory of the organism, health or disease—no unifying framework to tie it all together. Without a theory and a framework, there is no understanding of what the problems are, how they developed or how to solve them, and everything becomes an ad hoc experience. The mechanistic manner in which medicine is practiced today has never been proven by scientific method. As Lynne McTaggart, author of the 1996 book, *What Doctors Don't Tell You,* wrote: "For all the attempts to cloak medicine in the weighty mantle of science—a good deal of what we regard as standard medical practice today amounts to little more than 20th-century voodoo."

Doctors usually have little idea what is wrong with their patients or how to make them well. And how can one blame them? They spent many years in medical school, learning technicalities, procedures and protocols, and were taught that "cures" must come from outside the body. That is why physicians have no faith or instruction about the natural capacity of the human body to heal itself. In fact, many argue that almost all conditions presented to physicians are self-limiting and spontaneously resolve by the natural healing process, regardless of what the physician happens to prescribe.

This natural healing process must become our focus, because the magnitude of sickness in this country is astonishing. More than three out of four Americans now suffer from a diagnosable chronic disease, a dilemma that the modern medical establishment not only fails to solve, but actually contributes to. Things must change. In March 2001, The Institute of Medicine of the National Academy of Sciences issued a report titled, *Crossing the Quality Chasm: A New Health System for the 21st Century.* According to this report: ". . . between the health care we now have and the health care we could have lies not just a gap, but a chasm." The report also said: "Health care harms patients too frequently and routinely fails to deliver its potential benefits."

The United States has the most expensive, yet one of the most inadequate health care systems in the world. Our infant mortality rate is worse than Cuba's. According to the World Health Organization, our overall health is worse than that of almost every European country, as well as Australia, Canada, and Israel. According to the above Institute of Medicine report, ". . . a fundamental, sweeping redesign of the entire health care system is required." The report cited that ". . . the nation's health care delivery system has fallen short in its ability to translate knowledge into practice and to apply new technology safely and appropriately." It went on to say, ". . . if the system cannot consistently deliver today's science and technology, it is even less prepared to respond to the extraordinary advances that surely will emerge during the coming decades."

We've spent hundreds of billions of medical research dollars on outmoded science, which explains why we have not found the cause or the cure for a single chronic disease. Decades after President Richard Nixon declared "war on cancer" and after countless billions of dollars spent, malignancy survival rates are not noticeably improved. We have yet to produce a truly effective cancer treatment; every minute another American dies of cancer. The situation is similar with heart disease. We can implant a new artificial heart surgically, but we cannot prevent or cure heart disease. Why? Because so few resources are devoted to study of the body's healing systems or to help patients understand and support their own health at the cellular level. Reallocating resources with these priorities in mind is the direction medicine must take if it is ever to be effective in reversing our epidemic of chronic disease.

Everyone Is Unique

Interested only in identifying symptoms, physicians do not listen to their patients. Patients are regarded as machines, similar to every other machine; doctors need not learn anything unique about individual people. A study reported in the December 1993 issue of *Internal Medicine News* found that 70 percent of patients were interrupted by their doctor within eighteen seconds after the patient began to describe their symptoms. As soon as the doctor has matched symptoms to a disease, treatments follow established protocols. Everyone with the same "disease" receives the same treatment.

Such procedures completely ignore one of the greatest scientific discoveries of the twentieth century: biochemical individuality. Two people with the same so-called disease may need different treatments because no two people's cells are malfunctioning for exactly the same reasons. Modern medicine does not teach physicians how to recognize or work with each patient's unique biochemistry.

Even when presented with scientific evidence that an alternative system works best, most physicians resist change and fail to apply these findings. Their disease-based focus interferes with the essence of what health care should be: the optimization of health at the cellular level based on a person's unique biochemistry and life circumstances.

Resistant to Change

Adopting a more rational system of medicine would result in an enormous reduction in health-care costs by eliminating hundreds of thousands of physicians and closing thousands of hospitals (not to mention the potential financial ruin of drug companies). Obviously, the economic incentive to maintain the status quo and not change is enormous. Currently, cancer is a billion-dollar-a-day "industry" in the United States, and more people are employed in the AIDS industry than there are sufferers of AIDS.

Modern medicine's efforts to protect money and jobs were vividly described and documented in the 2000 book by former New York State Legislator, Daniel Haley, *Politics in Healing: The Suppression and Manipulation of American Medicine.* Haley points out that in the twentieth century several inexpensive and highly effective cures for cancer were introduced in American medicine. The developers of these cures, well-meaning people, were naive and believed that the world would welcome a cancer cure. What these people—among others, Harry Hoxey, William Frederick Koch, Royal Raymond Rife and Dr. Andrew Ivy—all failed to understand is that someone who threatens the survival of a prospering and growing industry with an inexpensive cure will not be welcomed. Proven and effective cancer cures were repudiated and suppressed by the American Medical Association (AMA) and the U.S. Food and Drug Administration (FDA). Discoverers of these cures were isolated, harassed, persecuted, prosecuted, financially ruined and destroyed, and their treatments essentially have been lost. Some events described in Haley's book are bizarre and are hard to believe, yet they are documented by evidence presented at jury trials and recorded in court records. The FDA, AMA, the National Cancer Institute, and the American Cancer Society still continue to suppress cancer cures, such as that developed by Dr. Stanislaw Burzynski; his office has been raided by FDA agents and U.S. Marshals, he has been persecuted relentlessly, and his medical license is on a ten-year probation during which time he is not allowed to see new patients. These actions prevent public access to treatments and intimidate other unorthodox physicians.

Physicians who have worked all their lives within the existing system often feel threatened by change. The majority of physicians support efforts by state medical boards and government regulatory boards to suppress alternative approaches. A less expensive, more effective way of practicing medicine threatens their economic well-being, as well as philosophically questions the validity of their lifetime work. Physicians who have dared to introduce alternative treatments have had their licenses revoked, been financially ruined, and ostracized because they were willing to help patients with treatments that were not the "accepted standard of care."

A chilling example of how nonconforming doctors are kept in line is the case of Jonathan Wright, M.D. On May 6, 1992, a small army of FDA agents plus ten police officers, with drawn guns and flak jackets, attacked Dr. Wright's office. Rather than simply opening the office door and walking in, they broke it down, terrifying his staff and patients in the waiting room. Why? Was Wright on the FBI's list of known terrorists? No. Wright was merely an outspoken critic of

modern medicine and the FDA, and he regularly used vitamins and natural substances in his practice. This approach to
healing made him a target.

During the fourteen-hour raid, all of Wright's records,
equipment, manuals, vitamins, minerals and herbs were con-
fiscated. They even took his postage stamps. None of Wright's
patients ever had complained about him. Wright was never
charged with anything, nor ever prosecuted for anything. Yet,
both his practice and his reputation were damaged. It took
years and hundreds of thousands of dollars in legal fees to
have his patient records returned and his practice restored.
Events like this are not supposed to happen in America, but
they do happen to doctors who step out of line. As a result, we
are denied the right to choose certain treatments because our
doctors cannot offer them.

Most people are unaware that a physician can lose his or her
license to practice by failing to adhere to "prevailing standards
of practice in their community." A loss of license can occur
even if no patient is harmed, no patient has complained and
the condition of the patients involved actually improved.
Physicians can learn something new at a medical conference
or from a medical journal, but they cannot use it in their practice. The only treatments allowed are the ones already in use,
which makes innovation and progress slow to almost impossible. Physicians must be very courageous to depart from traditional practices, even if they believe doing so can be helpful.

Money is at stake, and competition from less expensive,
natural treatments is discouraged. The FDA is supposed to
regulate drugs to assure that they are safe and effective. In
practice, FDA-approved, properly prescribed drugs kill about
four hundred people every day. Why? Because the FDA has
become an instrument of the pharmaceutical companies. The
drug industry is among the most profitable in the world, and
Americans pay more for the same drugs than people in other
countries. To help protect these economic interests, about

one-half of the senior officials at the FDA formerly were employed as key executives in the drug industry. After leaving the FDA, about half eventually return to executive positions in drug companies. This practice is termed "the revolving door." The FDA is very biased in favor of drugs, and people are denied free access to the documented health benefits of nutritional supplements. Needless to say, these people are not in favor of treating diseases with vitamins. Both manufacturers and retailers of supplements have been subjected to FDA seizures and harassment.

One of the supposed justifications for modern medicine's suppression of alternative approaches is that they have not been properly tested for safety and effectiveness. In truth, many alternative approaches (such as the use of vitamin supplements) are supported by thousands of sound studies, while, ironically, up to 90 percent of the techniques and procedures used by modern medicine have never been proven to be safe or effective.

Medical Malpractice

According to a 1995 issue of the *Journal of the American Medical Association,* more than 1 million people per year are injured in hospitals, and 180,000 die from those injuries. Illnesses caused by prescription drugs are estimated to cost more than $136 billion a year. A 1981 study published in the *New England Journal of Medicine* concluded that at least one-third of hospital patients suffered some ill effect during their stay, and that 9 percent suffered major injury. Consider what the late Robert Mendelsohn, M.D., author of the 1979 book *Confessions of a Medical Heretic,* wrote: "I believe that more than ninety percent of Modern Medicine could disappear from the face of the earth—doctors, hospital, drugs, and equipment—and the effect on our health would be immediate and beneficial."

Normally, one might think that if doctors went on strike the public would suffer serious health problems. Yet, Mendelsohn noted cases when doctors went on strike and the death rate declined. In 1973, doctors were on strike in Israel for a month, and this coincided with a decline of 55 percent in the death rate. In 1976, a fifty-two-day doctor strike in Bógota, Colombia, coincided with a decline in mortality of 35 percent. The same year, in Los Angeles, doctors staged a slowdown, and the death rate dropped by 18 percent. In each case, when the doctors' labor actions ended, mortality rates shot back up to prior levels.

In recent years, a number of medical journals, such as *Pediatrics, Lancet, Annual Review of Public Health,* and particularly the July 26, 2000, *Journal of the American Medical Association,* have been filled with statistics on injuries and deaths caused by modern medical practice. The most recent annual estimate of hospital-caused deaths is:

- 106,000 deaths from "properly" prescribed drugs.
- 80,000 deaths from hospital-caused infections.
- 12,000 deaths from unnecessary surgery.
- 7,000 deaths from medication errors.
- 20,000 deaths from other errors.

These numbers total 225,000 deaths per year, but the real total is far greater. These numbers do not include unreported medically caused deaths. Why take responsibility for a death if another plausible explanation can be given? Even in good hospitals, only one "adverse event" out of four is reported; some studies have placed the reporting as low as one out of twenty. Medicine-caused deaths in outpatient settings have been estimated as an additional 200,000 per year. Again, this figure is conservative. Perhaps one of the biggest problems, though, is X rays.

The Threat of X Rays

One of the most serious threats to our health may be caused by one type of medical testing: medical and dental X rays. There is no safe radiation level; any amount of radiation can cause our cells to malfunction. The radiation levels from medical and dental X rays (though supposedly within "safe limits") contribute to both cancer and coronary heart disease. Evidence was published in 1999 by John Gofman, a medical doctor and a Ph.D. nuclear physicist, who is one of the world's leading authorities on radiation damage. Dr. Gofman's book, *Radiation from Medical Procedures in the Pathogenesis of Cancer and Ischemic Heart Disease,* presents a compelling argument for reconsidering how we understand disease and death rates in our society and modern medicine's responsibility for them. Gofman's research caused him to conclude that medical radiation was probably the single largest cause of cancer mortality in the twentieth century.

Gofman's evidence suggests that medical X rays are a necessary cofactor, meaning that while other factors are involved, the X ray is necessary for both cancer and heart disease to develop. Dr. Gofman found that more than 60 percent of deaths from cancer and more than 70 percent of deaths from coronary heart disease involved X rays. To cite just one example, Gofman found that in 1990, medical X rays were a necessary causal factor in 83 percent of all breast cancer. In other words, chest X rays and mammograms are the leading cause of breast cancer.

Fortunately, thermography is a safe and effective alternative to mammograms. Thermography measures temperature and appears to be a far more accurate way of detecting tumors at a much earlier stage. A cancerous tumor, as it begins to receive its own blood supply, is warmer than the surrounding tissue and can be discerned when the temperature of the breast is measured.

Modern medicine is responsible for about 90 percent of our

exposure to man-made radiation, and about 90 percent of that exposure is the result of diagnostic X rays. A level of radiation less than that produced by ten bitewing dental X rays can produce thyroid cancer, and not surprisingly, an epidemic of thyroid cancer is now being found in people who had upper chest, neck and head X rays decades ago.

Nevertheless, X rays are performed with alarming frequency. Gofman estimates that more than half are not necessary. Other researchers have placed the percentage of X rays of "little to no medical value" as high as 90 percent. Even low-level X rays are capable of inflicting genetic damage, presenting a hazard to both existing and future generations. For example, correlations have been found between the number of abdominal X rays a mother had received in her lifetime and the birth of a baby with Down's syndrome.

The public worries about radiation from nuclear power plants, yet a more common hazard is radiation from medical X rays. Decline X rays unless they are absolutely necessary, which is not often. Children are especially vulnerable to radiation and need to be protected by their parents.

Applying Dr. Gofman's data on medical X rays to 60 percent of the deaths from cancer and 70 percent of the deaths from ischemic heart disease in this country, I calculated that X rays cause about 650,000 deaths every year. Combining these deaths with the acknowledged number of medicine-caused deaths (250,000 inpatient and 200,000 outpatient per year) reveals an estimated total of more than 1 million deaths per year caused by modern medical practice. This figure amounts to about half of all deaths in America, making modern medicine our leading cause of death.

Should You Have Medical Testing?

Among the treatments that cause patients harm are diagnostic tests, everything from ultrasound to X rays, from blood tests to barium enemas. Many of these tests are inaccurate, present more risk than benefit and alternatives often are safer and more effective. The only time these tests are justified are when safety is clearly in question and only when the results of the test would require action. Avoid tests that simply provide information. For example, avoid ultrasounds during pregnancy, which do little more than inform parents about their child's development and rarely lead to any meaningful action.

Always question your doctor carefully about whether a particular medical test is necessary, especially if the test is invasive. All tests need not be avoided, but ask about potential risks as well as benefits. Be aware that most doctors downplay risks. Remember, a diagnostic test precipitated my own health crisis.

Most often doctors order tests to measure symptoms in order to make a diagnosis. Such testing is not especially useful because it is not designed to measure the causes of disease: deficiency and toxicity. Doctors should be ordering tests that measure, directly or indirectly, levels of deficiency and toxicity and what is causing them. If the tests are not for these purposes, they may be unnecessary. Many diagnostic tests are ordered solely for defensive purposes, so that physicians can prove they considered every possibility in the event of legal action. Decline tests if the doctor is unable to explain how it will help to measure and correct your cellular deficiency and toxicity.

Every invasive test poses some risk. Even a simple blood test poses the danger of an infection developing at the puncture site. Punctures for removal of fluid from the joints, bone, spinal column and womb pose greater risks. Be especially wary of signing an informed consent for a diagnostic test, tip-off about the degree of risk involved.

If the accuracy of test results seems questionable, seek a second opinion. Be skeptical of any diagnosis based solely on a test. If something is found abnormal and the doctor wants to

prescribe, request to have the test repeated before doing something that could cause damage, be it needless surgery, biopsies, medications, anxiety or financial cost. Suppose that a
particular medical test is 95 percent accurate. For every
twenty tests given, one false result will occur, usually a false
positive. If a person has this test twenty times in a lifetime, the
odds are in favor of at least one false result. In fact, many diseases can be "cured" simply by redoing the test. In 1975, the
Centers for Disease Control and Prevention surveyed medical
testing labs nationally and concluded that more than 25 percent of all test results were wrong; for certain clinical chemistry tests, the error rate was 50 percent. Not a lot has changed
since then.

A study in the May 1997 issue of *Hippocrates* examined
169 different kinds of medical diagnostic tests and concluded
that only nine of them actually did anything for the patient for
reducing the incidence of disease. According to the article,
many of these tests regularly led to faulty diagnoses, resulting
in unnecessary treatments the patients did not need, and
people with passing chest or back pain were "being marched
off to surgery to get their hearts repaired or spines fixed."

About 70 percent of all pregnant American women undergo
ultrasound evaluations, yet studies published in medical journals including *Lancet* and the *Canadian Medical Association
Journal* show that ultrasound may affect fetal growth, resulting in babies with lower birth weight. In addition, children are
twice as likely to have delayed speech development if they
were examined via ultrasound as a fetus. A 1995 study done at
the Massachusetts Institute of Technology and reported in
Science found that low-frequency ultrasound increases the
permeability of human skin, allowing proteins to pass through
more easily. Ultrasound definitely affects the body's tissues,
yet it is presented to patients as a procedure free of risks and
side effects.

Should You Have Surgery?

Modern surgery certainly is one of the crowning achievements in modern medicine. Surgery works very well to correct physical problems, such as those sustained in accidents, sports injuries and from birth defects, but surgery does not solve disease problems. Unfortunately, most surgery is performed to address disease problems, wasting resources and permanently damaging the patient. Every part of the human body is important to the functioning of the whole; removing malfunctioning body parts does not solve the real problem. Surgery should not be performed unless there is absolutely no alternative, and there is almost always an alternative.

Most conventional cancer treatments—especially surgery—are directed by the mechanistic belief system described earlier. Cancer is regarded as affecting a specific location or body part that should be removed physically or otherwise poisoned and killed. Completely forgotten is that cancer is a systemic disease affecting the entire body, and that a sounder approach is to restore cancerous cells to normal by addressing their deficiency and toxicity.

Cancer patients who properly address their deficiency and toxicity may experience what is termed "spontaneous remission." A study by Dr. Harold Foster at the University of British Columbia in 1988 found that virtually every one of two hundred cancer patients who had experienced a spontaneous cancer remission had actually done something to improve their cell chemistry. Eighty-seven percent had made major changes to their diet, while others had used nutritional supplements and detoxification programs. Currently, numerous alternative treatments for cancer are available (see appendix D).

A heart bypass operation is another example of unnecessary surgery. In 1992, Nortin Hadler, M.D., a professor of medicine at the University of North Carolina Medical School, concluded that 95 to 97 percent of the coronary bypass surgeries done that year were unnecessary—even though patients usually are told that without the surgery they will die. In truth, almost all coronary disease is preventable with diet, supplements and exercise. Likewise, coronary disease is reversible, as pioneers like Nathan Pritikin, more recently Dean Ornish, M.D., and others, have proven.

How much surgery is necessary? Dr. Robert Mendelsohn, in *Confessions of a Medical Heretic,* said, "My feeling is that somewhere around ninety percent of surgery is a waste of time, money, energy, and life." Dr. Mendelsohn cites an independent review of people recommended for surgery. The study found that most of these patients did not need surgery and half of them needed no medical treatment at all. In another case, a hospital oversight committee reviewed surgically removed tissues. In the year prior to the formation of the committee, the hospital performed 262 appendectomies—after the committee was formed, the number dropped to 62. The committee found that most of the tissues being removed were healthy! In March 1997, the Physicians Committee for Responsible Medicine published a statement saying that only 10 percent of hysterectomies are justified. In addition to being almost entirely unnecessary, surgery is risky; possibilities exist for surgical error, complications from anesthesia and infection, not to mention the physical, mental and emotional shock to the body.

Should You Take Medicine?

All drugs have potentially damaging "side effects." Because a malfunctioning cell is the definition of disease, and drugs deliberately cause cells to malfunction, drugs cause disease. Drugs are foreign to the body; the mechanism by which drugs work is to alter the body's biochemistry in order to suppress symptoms. Side effects often are worse than the diseases the drugs are used to treat. Perhaps these hazards would be justified if drugs cured disease, but they do not, they control and suppress symptoms. Even with symptoms suppressed, the true cause of the problem may be growing worse while the body's natural healing mechanisms are being compromised by the drugs.

Billions of dollars are spent in the war against street drugs, but the number of people killed and injured by street drugs is minor compared to prescription drugs. Prescription drugs kill a couple of hundred thousand people every year and are a leading cause of disease and death. If your doctor prescribes a drug, consider that it may cause your cells to malfunction, and that alternatives exist that are both safe and effective.

Even aspirin and other common over-the-counter drugs are dangerous, so find alternatives that work for you. Books such as *Alternative Medicine: The Definitive Guide,* edited by the Burton Goldberg Group, and *Finding the Right Treatment,* by Jacqueline Krohn, M.D., and Francis Taylor, M.A., are excellent resources for those wishing to find natural alternatives to toxic prescription drugs.

Unfortunately, when drugs cause disease, we have all been trained not to call it disease. Instead, we use the deceptive term "side effects." In 1984, the drug industry attempted to obtain a legal exemption from the liability laws that apply to virtually all manufacturers. Why? Because even the people who make the drugs know they are not safe; "all prescription drugs are unavoidably unsafe" argued the Pharmaceutical Manufacturers Association. Of course, this wording is not used in drug advertisements aimed at the public.

A hospital patient receives, on average, twelve different drugs. Yet, often when as few as three are prescribed, absolutely no one understands all the dangerous interactions between the drugs. Bad enough taken one at a time, combinations of drugs can be particularly toxic. Prescription drugs are notorious for causing many adverse effects in the elderly, including memory loss, depression, confusion, constipation, Parkinson's disease, falls and urinary incontinence. All too often, a second drug is prescribed to suppress the symptoms caused by the first, then another to suppress the symptoms of the first two, and so forth. Many illnesses of the elderly really are manifestations of adverse drug reactions. A 1991 study in the *Journal of the American Medical Association* showed that 14 percent of in-hospital cardiac arrests followed a complication, usually because of a medication. Well-known combinations of commonly prescribed drugs can kill, and alert pharmacists have saved many lives.

Up to 29 percent of all hospital admissions are caused by adverse reactions to drugs, according to a 1995 study in the *Archives of Internal Medicine*. Many reactions result in liver damage, long hospital stays, permanent disability and even death. In 1990, an estimated 659,000 Americans aged sixty years and older were hospitalized due to adverse drug reactions. In addition to toxicity, drugs also can cause deficiency by depleting the body of essential nutrients. Diuretics cause excessive loss of potassium and other essential minerals. Anticonvulsants cause loss of vitamin D. Antibiotics, nonsteroidal anti-inflammatory drugs and steroid hormones can indirectly cause numerous vitamin and mineral deficiencies by causing digestive damage. Because of the complexity of the human organism, predicting the effects of drugs in each individual, especially with combinations of drugs, is impossible. Other facts:

- A January 1997 study in the *Journal of the American Medical Association* stated that drug-related morbidity and mortality costs more than $136 billion a year—more than the cost of cardiovascular disease, our leading cause of death.
- In 1995, Duke University researchers showed that drugs commonly prescribed for stroke patients actually hampered their recovery. Even after a single dose, the negative effects could be long-lasting.

- A 1994 study in the *Journal of the American Medical Association* concluded that inappropriate and potentially dangerous drugs are prescribed for one in four older Americans every year.
- A 1994 study published in the *Journal of the National Cancer Institute* and *The Journal of the Federation of American Societies for Experimental Biology* warned that antihistamine and antidepressant drugs (including Prozac) contain chemicals known to accelerate tumor growth. While these drugs do not cause cancer directly, they can speed its growth.

Three Classes of Common Drugs Are of Special Concern

Nonsteroidal anti-inflammatory drugs (NSAIDs): NSAIDs include over-the-counter drugs such as aspirin, ibuprofen and acetaminophen, and prescription drugs such as Indocin, Feldene, Naprosyn and others. Use of NSAIDs is a significant national health problem, causing long-term damage to large numbers of people, particularly the elderly, who are the largest users of these drugs. According to data published in *Hospital Practice* in December 1996, up to two hundred thousand Americans are hospitalized every year for problems caused by NSAIDs, and as many as twenty thousand people a year die from the damage.

NSAIDs usually are prescribed for a noble purpose, to relieve pain, and they are among the most commonly prescribed pharmaceuticals in the world. About 60 million NSAID prescriptions are written every year in America, and an estimated 14 million people take these drugs for symptomatic relief of arthritis alone. These drugs relieve pain, but at a cost. About one third of chronic NSAID users experience noticeable gastrointestinal discomfort, which is only the tip of the iceberg, indicating that digestive damage is occurring. In most people, NSAID-inflicted damage to the digestive system is asymptomatic (no obvious symptoms to warn of the damage being done). By the time the stomach or gut is in pain from NSAIDs, massive damage has already occurred.

Most physicians think it is acceptable for people to take NSAIDs, believing that they cause minimal and acceptable damage. Virtually everyone who takes these dangerous drugs has their health damaged, and the longer they are taken, the worse it becomes. People who take NSAIDs for arthritis for years suffer worse joint damage than those who take nothing. NSAIDs have been linked to kidney failure, cognitive dysfunction, hearing loss, ringing in the ears, macular degeneration and hormone disruption. Examples include:

- In a 1992 study published in the *Scandinavian Journal of Rheumatology,* long-term NSAID users were hospitalized six times more often than nonusers. Deaths from gastrointestinal causes occurred twice as often, and half of all patients who died of ulcer-related complications had reported recent use of NSAIDs.
- A 1996 study in the *Archives of Internal Medicine* found that patients taking NSAIDs were four to seventeen times more likely to suffer acute kidney failure.
- A 1996 study in *Physiological Behavior* showed NSAIDs interfere with melatonin production, with a 75 percent nighttime reduction. Decreased melatonin production has been associated with sleep disorders as well as promotion of cancer.
- A 1996 study in *Lancet* showed that aspirin, in any form, such as buffered or coated, causes gastrointestinal bleeding. As few as one aspirin can cause bleeding.

NSAIDs cause intestinal bleeding by blocking action of messenger molecules called prostaglandins. Some prostaglandins cause inflammation and pain, and others stimulate healing and repair. NSAIDs block both types. Because the intestinal lining is renewed very rapidly (about every three days), blocking the repair process results in a gut that is weak, inflamed and leaky.

What should you do for a headache? Simple acupressure techniques and homeopathic remedies work quite well. What should you do for pain or inflammation? Eat a whole-foods diet, at least 75 percent raw. Avoid sugar, white flour, hydrogenated oils, junk foods and colas, and drink plenty of pure water. Avoid meat and dairy, but choose oily fish such as salmon (ocean harvested, rather than farmed). Take vitamin C up to bowel tolerance, 2 to 4 grams of quercitin per day, 30 to 60 mg of zinc daily, 100,000 units of beta-carotene for several days, and then 25,000 for several weeks, plus vitamin A and vitamin E. Essential fatty acid supplements also are critical. Digestive enzymes help, and especially take 1 to 3 grams of bromelain or papain per day. A number of herbs as well as homeopathic remedies are anti-inflammatory. These are excellent alternatives to NSAIDs.

Antibiotics: Most of us have been given an antibiotic at one time or another, and this contributes to one of our largest sources of toxins—those generated within our own digestive systems. Antibiotics are designed to kill disease-causing bacteria, but they also kill the friendly bacteria in our digestive systems. If these bacteria are absent or out of balance, a chain of unhealthy events is initiated, including undigested or malabsorbed food. Beneficial intestinal bacteria produce needed vitamins, such as B-complex vitamins, vitamin B_{12} and vitamin K. These essential nutrients are no longer produced when the friendly bacteria are displaced, and vitamin deficiency can result.

In addition, friendly bacteria prevent undesirable yeasts from proliferating by competing for food and producing biotin to inhibit yeast growth. When antibiotics kill beneficial bacterial, undesirable yeasts and bacteria thrive and take over, establishing their own ecosystem. This inhibits the beneficial bacteria from reestablishing themselves. Yeasts also produce numerous immune-reactive substances that force the immune system to form antibodies constantly. This stress may lead to impaired functioning of the immune system to the point of immune suppression or even breakdown. Also, yeasts inhibit magnesium absorption (which can lead to numerous neurological problems), damage gut tissue and cause leaking gut syndrome. A variety of health problems can result, ranging from chronic fatigue to allergies, arthritis and other immune dysfunction diseases.

A January 1996 article in *Internal Medicine World Report* stated that in 1991, more than 40 million prescriptions were written in America for antibiotics to treat people for the common cold. This use is inappropriate; antibiotics have no effect on the common cold. Vast overprescribing of this type fosters the development of antibiotic-resistant bacteria.

In May 1996, the World Health Organization (WHO) issued a report warning that "incurable" strains of bacteria are being discovered. Many infectious diseases, formerly controllable with antibiotics, are reappearing in forms difficult or even impossible to treat. "We are standing on the brink of a global crisis in infectious diseases," said Hiroshi Nakajima, M.D., WHO's director general. The report warns that the spread of untreatable infections is threatening to undermine modern advances in health care. In many hospitals, antibiotic-resistant staphylococcus infections are epidemic. More and more people die every year from antibiotic-resistant infections, acquired in hospitals. The WHO report noted that the "inappropriate use of antibiotics" is to blame both for the increase in drug-resistant microbes and for the weakened immune systems of patients. Either factor is serious; combined, they are catastrophic. Weakened immune systems play a crucial role in the development of AIDS, autoimmune diseases, asthma, allergies and a long list of other health problems.

Antibiotics represent what may be the single most damaging

category of drugs employed by allopathic medicine, and, like most drugs, are unnecessary. Only sick people get sick; prevent infections by eating a good diet and avoiding toxins. Stay away from immune-damaging foods like sugar, take high-quality supplements, reduce stress and get regular exercise. If an infection does occur, natural remedies should be considered before defaulting to the antibiotics that physicians will undoubtedly prescribe. Take lots of vitamins A, C (up to the point where you begin getting excessive gas or diarrhea, then decrease), and E, garlic, herbs like echinacea, or homeopathic remedies. Natural antibiotics like olive leaf extract are also helpful.

Hormones: Hormones are critical to health because they are part of the body's self-regulating system. They control gene expression, and, as part of the body's vital communication systems, they help balance the body. Hormone chemistry is awesomely complex and when you begin tampering with it, the effects on the body's system of checks and balances are unknown and potentially catastrophic. Even minute hormone quantities can have a profound effect on the body. The human body manufactures only 50 to 100 millionths of a gram per day of thyroid hormone, resulting in a blood concentration of only one part per ten billion (1 in 10,000,000,000). Yet this minute amount has a major regulatory effect. Supplemental hormones are dangerous meddling in the unknown because it is so easy to interfere with the body's system of hormonal checks and balances. Prescription hormones—birth control pills, hormone replacement therapy and steroid hormones— are the most common threats, as are steroids found in over-the-counter products such as cortisone ointments and DHEA (dehydroepiandrosterone).

Hormones are part of the body's cell-to-cell communications system, helping the body to regulate. For instance, hormones are used to regulate blood sugar, which normally stays within narrow limits to keep the body, and especially the brain, supplied with the correct amount. If blood sugar is too high, the pancreas secretes insulin, which signals the cells to take up glucose, thus lowering blood sugar and returning to normal. If blood sugar drops too low, the pancreas secretes glucagon, which signals the liver to break down glycogen into glucose to raise blood sugar. In this way, different hormones act in pairs like a thermostat, turning systems on and off. This chemistry presents a delicate balancing act. All the hormones interact with each other in ways modern science is only beginning to understand. In blood-sugar regulation alone, at least six hormones are involved.

Steroid hormones are being prescribed almost as frequently as antibiotics, for allergic reactions, asthma, eczema, arthritis, ulcerative colitis, and for all types of inflammatory and autoimmune diseases. Often steroids are given to babies and children to alleviate inflammations of all kinds. Steroids can cause permanent and devastating damage, even after a single dose; once the body is thrown out of its natural self-regulatory mode, it sometimes never "gets back." Steroids' beneficial effects appear to decline in time, leaving patients in worse condition than before they started.

Steroids appear to be a "miracle cure" for asthma or arthritis; however, they merely suppress the symptoms of these conditions. They may make people feel better, but this feeling comes at a high price. The medical journals are filled with steroid-inflicted horror stories, such as osteoporosis, retarded child growth and vision loss:

- The *Annals of Internal Medicine* in November 1993 reported that after just four months of use, oral steroids can cause osteoporosis, with an 8 percent reduction in bone mass.
- The *British Medical Journal* in August 1994 reported that extensive eye damage and visual loss can be caused by

using topical, over-the-counter, 1 percent hydrocortisone ointment for two weeks.

- *Lancet* has reported that after only six weeks of use, inhaled steroids prescribed for asthma retard growth in children.

Alternative approaches to steroids include, for example, vitamin C and quercitin. These two natural anti-inflammatories accomplish similar results, but without the side effects. Whether one takes steroids orally, inhales them or rubs them on the skin doesn't matter; damage can be caused quickly and irreversibly. Rubbing a little cortisone ointment on the skin affects the chemistry of the entire body. Steroids taken during pregnancy can cause a child to suffer from autism and impaired cognitive performance. Topical and inhaled steroids can cause glaucoma and cataracts. Other reported problems include fluid retention, thinning skin, slowness in healing, headaches, muscle weakness, immune suppression, angina, hair loss and depression.

Over-the-counter hormones such as melatonin and DHEA are special problems, partly because they are so easy to obtain. Daily doses of 50 milligrams of DHEA have been linked to acne, oily skin, excessive facial hair growth in women and mood changes such as irritability and aggressiveness. DHEA is a steroid hormone with a molecular structure quite similar to cortisone. (Cortisone, too, was once thought to be a wonder drug, until we found it was maiming and killing people.) In a 1997 study conducted at Northwestern University, sixteen rats fed DHEA for eighteen months experienced color changes in their livers from pink to brown. Fourteen developed liver cancer.

Neurologists and other sleep specialists have warned against taking melatonin supplements. In September 1996, the National Institutes of Health sponsored a meeting in Bethesda, Maryland, where researchers reported that we do not have sufficient knowledge about how melatonin works to predict all its potential adverse effects, especially at the high doses in over-the-counter preparations. The data showed melatonin could cause nausea, headaches, nightmares, worsening of existing depression or a drop in body temperature, which increases the risk of developing viral infections. Richard J. Wurtman, M.D., professor of neuroscience and director of the clinical research center at the Massachusetts Institute of Technology, described widespread use of over-the-counter melatonin as "scary."

The original experiments with mice, suggesting that melatonin prolonged life, used genetically selected mice that were unable to produce melatonin. When given some melatonin, they did measurably better than having none. However, repeated experiments with normal mice resulted in shortened life span, because they developed tumors of the reproductive tract. (Of course, the public hears only of the "benefits.")

Taking hormones on a regular basis, such as the numerous women on birth control pills and others on hormone replacement therapy (HRT), imbalances the hormone system. Millions of women are put on HRT, presumably to help prevent heart attack and osteoporosis. Little reliable evidence exists that HRT prevents either; in fact evidence shows that it promotes these conditions.

Want to prevent hormone disruption in your body? Avoiding certain toxins is critical. More than fifty different chemicals are known to disrupt the normal communication jobs of hormones, including pesticides, PCBs and dioxins, phthalates leached from PVC and other plastics, and bisphenol-A (from polycarbonate water bottles and the plastics used to coat the interior of cans used to contain food). Dietary considerations are important, because most of our exposure to these hormone-disrupting chemicals comes from eating meat and dairy products. Sugar and white flour disrupt hormone balances, so minimize consumption. Rest and exercise help balance hormone levels; moderate exercise doubles or even quadruples beneficial growth hormone levels. Most critically, our society must stop such constant and widespread use of hormone drugs. As John Mills, M.D., chief of infectious diseases at San Francisco General Hospital said, steroid hormones are "probably the most sleazy of modern-day medications."

Digestive Destruction

As you know, one way in which drugs cause disease is by interfering with the digestion of food and absorption of nutrients. By damaging gut tissue, killing off beneficial bacteria, and creating an environment that inhibits the growth of normal, beneficial gut bacteria, we lose our ability to digest food and absorb nutrients properly. This condition creates both deficiency and toxicity, the two causes of cellular malfunction and disease.

Three classes of drugs are responsible for much of this damage: NSAIDs, antibiotics and hormones. NSAIDs physically damage gut tissue and destabilize the normal composition of bacteria living in the gut, especially if combined with antibiotics. Antibiotics kill friendly bacteria essential to health and result in a variety of intestinal infections. Hormones, such as birth control pills, create chemical imbalances in the gut, thus promoting yeast infections such as candida. Once yeasts change the environment in the digestive system, a long chain of events damage health and cause disease.

Gut tissue that is damaged becomes more permeable ("leaky") to large molecules of undigested food and to microorganisms that enter the bloodstream and circulate throughout the body. This occurrence provokes chronic immune responses manifested as food allergies and other inflammatory conditions, and such inflammatory conditions may be the basis of all chronic disease.

These immune responses sometimes create antibodies that match certain body tissues and attack them, resulting in autoimmune diseases such as lupus or arthritis. A person who has a damaged gut may eat an excellent diet but still suffer malnutrition because of nutrient malabsorption.

Adding malabsorption to an already deficient diet is catastrophic to long-term health. Excessive immune reactions produce much debris, called immune complexes, which can overburden the kidneys and cause kidney disease. In fact, allergic reactions may be the leading cause of kidney disease. Major and uncorrected maldigestion can lead to extreme weight loss and greater susceptibility to opportunistic infections, commonly experienced in people with AIDS.

Vaccinations

Popular opinion regards vaccinations as one of modern medicine's greatest achievements, preventing more suffering and saving more lives than any other medical procedure. Nothing could be further from the truth. Any risks or "side effects" from vaccinations supposedly far outweigh the inherent benefits. However, finding benefits is difficult and finding risks is easy.

You have a better chance of being healthy if your cells are healthy; vaccinations damage your cells. In fact, modern medicine's practice of mass vaccinations may be a blunder that ranks with X rays and antibiotics for damage done to health. No reliable safety study has ever been performed on any vaccine, and evidence suggests that they are both ineffective and harmful. Yet, individuals are forced, without consent, to risk injury or even death.

In October 2000, at the annual meeting of the Association of American Physicians and Surgeons (AAPS), a resolution called for an end to all government-mandated vaccinations. Even more astounding, the resolution passed without a single dissenting vote. Jane Orient, M.D., executive director of the AAPS, said, "Our children face the possibility of death or serious long-term adverse effects from mandated vaccines that aren't necessary or that have limited benefits." The AAPS's resolution read that "mass vaccination is equivalent to human experimentation and subject to the Nuremberg Code, which requires voluntary informed consent." By failing to inform us of the dangers, and taking away our power to choose otherwise, mandated vaccinations become a crime against humanity.

The dramatic decline of infectious diseases, such as smallpox, diphtheria and polio, often is cited (inaccurately) as proof of vaccinations' effectiveness. The incidence of infectious disease dramatically decreased *before* the introduction of vaccines; in other words, vaccines get credit for something they did not do. In 1950, the polio epidemic was at its height in Great Britain. By the time polio vaccine was introduced in 1956, polio had already declined by 82 percent. Similarly, tuberculosis was a persistent killer throughout the 1800s and by 1945 had already declined by 97 percent. Other infectious diseases that already were in decline before the introduction of their vaccines include pneumonia, influenza, whooping cough and measles. Continuing decline merely followed the existing trend. *Countries that did not vaccinate against specific diseases experienced similar declines as countries that did.*

A strong argument for the decline of infectious diseases can be made for a variety of factors, including better sanitation, less crowded living conditions and the absence of hunger. In addition, diseases tend to have their own evolutionary cycles; they go away as the population gains "herd" immunity. Diseases like bubonic plague and scarlet fever experienced declines similar to other infectious diseases; they disappeared without any immunization programs.

Finding any studies that prove vaccines' effectiveness is difficult. To prove efficacy, we must analyze studies of vaccinated groups versus unvaccinated ones. Very few of such studies ever have been conducted; the few that have been indicate that the vaccines are ineffective. Recent worldwide outbreaks of virulent forms of TB have demonstrated that alleged "protection" by TB vaccine has little to do with whether or not anyone contracts the disease.

Not only ineffective, vaccines can also be harmful. Viera Scheibner, Ph.D., a world authority on immunizations and author of the 1993 book *Vaccination,* wrote: "Immunizations . . . not only did not prevent any infectious diseases, they caused more suffering and more deaths than any other human activity in the entire history of medical intervention." Having assembled and researched the world's largest collection of data on immunizations, Dr. Scheibner concludes that "there is no evidence whatsoever that vaccines of any kind— but especially those against childhood diseases—are effective in preventing the infectious diseases they are supposed to prevent. . . . One hundred years of orthodox research shows that vaccines represent a medical assault on the immune system."

Each generation is subjected to more vaccinations and, as a result, is experiencing more immune dysfunction diseases. Many children have as many as twenty-two vaccinations before they go to the first grade, and as more vaccines become available, the number keeps increasing. At an international conference in 1997, Terry Phillips, Ph.D., D.Sc., professor of medicine at George Washington University Medical Center, reported that the foreign proteins in virtually all vaccines wreak havoc on the human immune system. Vaccines are toxic mixtures loaded with various substances that never should be injected into a human body—including foreign proteins and dangerous viruses from chickens, guinea pigs, calves and monkeys. Some researchers believe these viruses put a permanent burden on our immune systems and do continuous damage both to the immune and nervous systems. Vaccines also contain toxic chemicals, like mercury (a neurotoxin), ethylene glycol (antifreeze), formaldehyde (a carcinogen), aluminum (a carcinogen and also associated with Alzheimer's), plus antibiotics like Streptomycin (which can cause allergic reactions). Even the FDA has called for cessation of mercury in vaccines because our children are being exposed to unsafe amounts of it.

Dr. Harris Coulter, in his various writings on vaccinations, says that the allergic response initiated with an injected vaccine is capable of causing encephalitis (an inflammation of the brain). Encephalitis can cause permanent brain damage and lead to lifelong problems of autism, dyslexia, learning disabilities, behavioral disorders and antisocial syndromes. Dr. Coulter estimates that 50 percent of the children who experience a fever after vaccination actually are suffering from encephalitis; he blames vaccines for the "new morbidity" of learning disabilities and behavioral disorders.

Decisions about whether to be vaccinated before a trip to a foreign country, or whether to vaccinate your children, should be based on accurate information. Unfortunately, the public has had little access to research questioning the safety and effectiveness of vaccinations.

Compulsory vaccination laws exist in every state. However, there are legal exemptions. Learn what the exemptions are in your state and obtain an appropriate one. All states have a medical exemption that a doctor can sign, and many states have religious exemptions, which do not require affiliation with any specific religion.

Regarding the common flu shot, consider this study published in *Lancet:* Absenteeism of more than one hundred thousand employees was noted each winter for three years, and the conclusion was that flu shots did not confer any protection. What about tetanus? Probably the single most important factor in preventing tetanus is thorough cleansing of the wound by removing all foreign bodies and dead tissue. On rare occasion, "tetanus-prone" wounds might justify a booster vaccine for those individuals already immunized, and immune globulin in those who never have been vaccinated.

To avoid an infectious disease, you don't need to have vaccinations; you need to keep your immunity strong. From the beginning, breastfeeding protects against many infections. Avoid allergenic foods like milk and wheat. Allergies lower immunity and predispose the body to infections. Nutritional status is critical to immune competence. Refined sugars are well known to depress immunity. Regular exercise, a good diet, and avoidance of allergens and toxins help to maintain a healthy immune system. Moreover, a high-quality supplement program is essential.

Give Credit Where It Is Due

While a dramatic decline has occurred in mortality during the last century, this decline has little to do with the "advancement" of our health-care system. Researchers at Harvard University and Boston University have determined that drugs, vaccines and other medical measures contributed a mere 1 to 3.5 percent to the decline in U.S. mortality since the turn of the century. This data appeared in a 1977 article (published in the summer edition of the *Milbank Memorial Fund Quarterly*), which concluded that increased life expectancy was due to improvements in sanitation and living conditions rather than advances in medicine. That view was supported in a study reported in the September 1977 issue of the *Journal of the American Medical Association,* concluding that "the most dramatic improvements in the health of our people as a group have been from cleaning up the water supply: sanitation, not medical care." The decline in mortality is primarily attributable to the decline in killer epidemics such as tuberculosis, scarlet fever, smallpox, diphtheria and others. The development of city sewer systems, water purification systems, pasteurization, refrigeration and food hygiene have done far more to prevent infectious disease than all modern medical treatments combined.

Watch Out for Your Dentist, Too

Dentists contribute to toxic loads and chronic disease just like physicians do—primarily through the use of local anesthetics and toxic metals (mercury amalgams and metal crowns). Mercury amalgams have been in use for more than one hundred years, and we have always been told they are safe. A "silver" amalgam is actually 50 percent mercury, and this mercury does not stay only in your mouth; the mercury is absorbed by the body and poisons cells. Almost everyone knows that lead is toxic, and lead-based paints have been outlawed since the 1970s. No one would think of putting lead in their mouth and sucking on it twenty-four hours a day, yet mercury is five thousand times more toxic than lead, and dentists use it in amalgams as if it were harmless.

Since 1988, the Environmental Protection Agency has classified scrap dental amalgams as a hazardous waste. Putting amalgams down the drain or in the trash, or burying them in a landfill, is illegal—but the FDA still says they can be put in our mouths! Fortunately, things are changing. In 1992, the German government banned the sale and manufacture of dental amalgams. Metal crowns are another problem, and even "porcelain" crowns are usually made with nickel—a toxic metal and a known carcinogen.

If you already have these toxic metals imbedded in tooth tissue, consider having them removed but only by someone highly skilled in such removals. Gold is a high-quality metal, and the only one acceptable for the mouth, but even gold is not perfect because it is mixed with other metals to make it harder. While no perfect dental material is available, new plastic materials, when properly installed in fillings or as crowns, appear to be the most acceptable choices for now. As with all health-related problems, prevention is best. Eat a good diet, free of refined sugar, and be sure to brush and floss. Be particular about what type of toothpaste, too (see appendix C).

In addition to being toxic, putting different metals in the mouth in the presence of saliva, which is electrically conductive, generates subtle electrical currents that corrode the metals in the mouth. Once metals begin to corrode and degrade, they become biologically active and begin circulating around various bodily tissues, leading to toxic accumulation. In addition, the subtle electrical currents can also affect other body functions and cause numerous problems, including hearing loss, insomnia, and difficulties with memory and concentration.

Local anesthetics (including lidocaine) are commonly used by dentists and may be substantial contributors to our cancer epidemic. These anesthetics break down in the body into cancer-causing compounds called anilines. In 1993, the FDA found that lidocaine, when exposed to human tissue, breaks down into 2, 6-dimethylaniline, a compound that is known to cause virtually every kind of cancer in animals, and it does so more than 99 percent of the time. In September 1996, as a result of these findings, the FDA removed from the market all over-the-counter painkillers containing these local anesthetics and required that a warning be placed on all new prescription pharmaceuticals containing them. Unfortunately, existing prescription anesthetics were not required to carry the warning, and most health professionals are still unaware of this problem.

Work with your dentists and doctors to minimize exposure to local anesthetics. Local anesthetics are given more often than necessary—usually for the dentist's convenience. Use these products only when absolutely necessary, and use the minimum dose necessary. Do not keep requesting more anesthetic because of the fear of "not quite being numb." Alternatives include: acupuncture, hypnosis, rubbing oil of cloves on the gum.

The Healer Within Yourself

Regardless of which medical treatments you choose, understand how the treatments actually work and how they affect your cells. Treatments designed to optimize or balance the function of your cells generally are safer and more effective than treatments designed to mask symptoms. Take medicine only when you need it (you definitely want to question taking drugs every day as a part of life), and only after you have compared (and attained second opinions on) benefits and possible side effects. Remember that you are in charge and you must take responsibility for your own health by supporting your body's natural abilities to repair and regulate itself.

John Lee, M.D., wrote in his 1993 book, *Optimal Health Guidelines:* "Going to the doctor these days can be risky business. In generations past, the basic tenet of medical care was 'Primum non nocere' (above all, do no harm). Today that dictum has been modified to 'do as little harm as possible.' Even that . . . is becoming operationally impossible. The patient must now learn to look out for himself."

Physicians do have their place, but one has to know what that place is. For example, anyone with acute health problems, such as a stroke, a bleeding ulcer or chest pains, should seek immediate medical attention. However, people who are suffering from chronic disease problems (cancer, heart disease, diabetes, arthritis, high blood pressure, depression and so forth) are best advised to avoid modern conventional medicine and to seek competent alternative care. Traditional healers typically worked to balance the body, both physically and energetically, thereby promoting health. That remains the underlying approach of many alternative practitioners and alternative treatments, including a growing number of enlightened M.D.s, naturopaths, homeopaths, acupuncturists, chiropractors, energy healers, massage therapists and others.

Conventional medicine is a powerful moneymaking bureaucracy that is incredibly resistant to change, but there is also a growing movement in this country to pass medical freedom laws that would bring more competition and creativity into the medical marketplace. (Physicians would then be free to pursue treatments that are not only safe, but more effective, such as treating heart disease with diet and supplements rather than surgery; treating cancer with nutrition, detoxification and herbs; and treating stroke with hyperbaric oxygen.) About half of all patients in America now seek at least some form of alternative treatment; people are putting the power of health into their own hands. This statement shouldn't suggest that alternative treatments are always safe and effective—indeed, many are not—but the growing discontent with our conventional health-care system is a reality that we can no longer ignore. Optimizing your position on the *medical pathway* requires being aware of the hazards of modern medicine as well as its miracles. You, not your doctor, are responsible for your health.

11

A SHIFT IN PERSPECTIVE

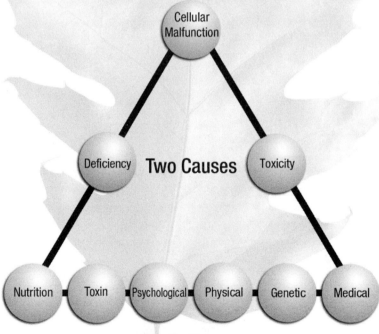

One Disease

Cellular Malfunction

Deficiency **Two Causes** Toxicity

Nutrition Toxin Psychological Physical Genetic Medical

Six Pathways

*"This pattern of high resistance and freedom from degener-
ative disease is seen wherever people live beyond the reach of
modern civilization and are not suffering from famine."*

Charles McGee, M.D.
How to Survive Modern Technology

P erspective is everything. By reshaping our understanding of disease, we are empowered to create
health. Are you ready to take charge of your health
and experience a state of well-being that even your doctors
may doubt is possible?

As you have read this book, you have discovered ways in
which you must change your life in order to get better and in
order to stay well. Perhaps you are fighting a disease with
little success, and now you see hope. Or perhaps you have
considered yourself "healthy," only to recognize that your
body already is showing early warning signs of disease.

Do you have a general feeling that your body is struggling
to keep up? Are you confused or frustrated by your medical
doctors or their recommended treatments? Are you distressed
by the number of prescription drugs or over-the-counter
medicines you take in order to keep going, even if you have no

sense you are getting better? Are you suffering a variety of symptoms that no doctor has been able to help you with? Are you making unhealthful choices in the foods that you eat, in the products that you use on yourself or in your home, and in other aspects of your life?

Before I got so sick and almost died in 1985, I lived a different life from the life I live today. I thought I was healthy and that I was living a healthful lifestyle; in reality I was encouraging sickness. I suffered from a number of diseases—allergies, colds, flu, tooth decay, joint pain, abdominal pain and fatigue. I went to physicians and dentists. I took antibiotics for infections, NSAIDs for pain and antihistamines for my allergies. I occasionally took vitamins, but I did so whimsically, without commitment and consistency, and certainly without a scientific understanding of which vitamins I should be taking and why. I ate most of my meals in upscale restaurants and spared no expense. My food choices, however, were based mostly on taste and enjoyment. I neither knew much nor thought much about nutrition.

When I did develop digestive problems and allergies, I was unaware that my food was causing the problems or that it would be possible to avoid them if I paid closer attention to what I ate. I am now aware of my allergy to dairy, but back then I ate ice cream, milk and other dairy products almost daily. I developed itchy eyes, mucus and sneezing fits after I ate them, but still I did not recognize the connection. I had grown accustomed to these "minor nuisances" and never imagined life could be so much better without them.

I used to eat far too much meat and dairy—at one or two meals every day—unaware that most of the pesticides we are exposed to have bioaccumulated in the animal products we consume. Although I don't recommend a meat-free diet, I recommend eating meat only a few times a week and only that which has been organically produced. The animal products I consumed back then contributed to my toxic load, as did the volumes of sugar, white flour and processed oils that were a regular part of my diet. In addition, both as a graduate research assistant at MIT and in my first job as a chemist, I was exposed to extraordinary amounts of toxic chemicals. Chemicals that are used today only in small amounts and with protective equipment we used to slosh around in the lab as if they were water. Back then, we were unaware of the full extent of their toxicity, and the manufacturers were in no rush to study the toxicities.

My discoveries about health and disease saved my life and changed my life—forever.

I learned to recognize which foods harmed my health. I learned to listen to my body's own warning signs. I learned how to avoid getting sick and how to accelerate recovery. I learned how to get well and stay well.

Since my recovery in 1987, I have rarely been sick. At age sixty-five, I have more energy, vitality and health than I did twenty years ago. I have taken no medications—neither a prescription drug nor an over-the-counter product—in the past seventeen years. Neither have I required the services of a physician in that time. I am no longer debilitated by my allergies. If I do get sick, I know what I can do to improve my situation. On the rare occasion that I do come down with a cold, I take plenty of high-quality vitamin C, and the cold vanishes in a matter of *hours* rather than after days or weeks of misery.

The lightning bolt that sparked these massive changes in my life and which guides my life today was a radical change in my perspective. I now see health as a choice, entirely within my control. I optimize my choices along all six pathways and I avoid disease. I shun "modern medicine," prescription drugs and other traditional treatments because I recognize that they treat the symptoms and not the causes of disease. Furthermore, modern medical treatments do harm.

Because I am able to keep my health in balance, I do not need drugs, medical treatments or doctors. I eat a wide variety of fresh organic foods, either from farmers' markets or health food stores. My favorites include apples, raw nuts and fresh vegetables used to make salads. I eat animal protein a few times per week, usually deep-water ocean fish (not farmed), organically produced poultry (without antibiotics and hormones) and organic eggs. I drink bottled water delivered in glass bottles. I supplement my diet with essential fatty acids and I avoid hydrogenated oils. On rare occasions I do have desserts, but even then I avoid common allergens like dairy. I definitely do not succumb to the daily after-dinner "sweet tooth." Refined sugar has been almost completely cut out of my life because it is so very dangerous. I avoid all corn and corn products because corn is now genetically contaminated as well as often being moldy. I minimize white potatoes and have completely eliminated french fries because they are one of the most toxic foods we eat. I take a variety of high-quality supplements, including amino acids (prior to meals), multivitamins, extra calcium/magnesium, vitamin E, quercitin and coenzyme Q10. I also take digestive enzymes with my meals.

In my home I have natural-fiber carpets, I have a filter on my shower to remove the chlorine, and I replaced my gas-fired water heater with an electric unit. On my body I use only toothpaste, shampoo and soap that do not have synthetic foaming agents, stabilizers, preservatives, colors or fragrances. For exercise I do daily rebounding, walking or hiking. During weekly visits to the gym, I do gentle weightlifting, treadmill, bicycling, and absolutely a sauna afterward to detoxify. I keep my spirits up by having purpose in my life, being excited about what I am doing and having people in my life that I care about. I teach as many as I can how to be healthy. All of the factors bring a sense of purpose and encouragement. I live in the present and in the future, and I do not dwell on the past. If I had only one day left to live, I would want to be excited about living that day.

Getting Sick Is Harder Than Staying Well

You may wonder if you have the ability, the energy and the resolve to make these kinds of life changes yourself. You do. But change is difficult, especially in the beginning. As I was reforming my life, I had to make a lot of adjustments. What I know for certain is that health problems are much harder to live with than these solutions. When I recognize that something I eat, something I do or something I expose myself to will make me sick, I simply do not want it anymore. It truly becomes that easy. You need to become a leader, however, as those around you may add pressure or distraction. If the people you live with or work with are eating unhealthful diets, you must be the one to set a different example.

People often ask me if I miss some of the "bad" things. No, I don't. Tastes change. New tastes can be acquired in a few weeks, and old ones can be lost. I used to love filet mignon, but after not eating it for ten years, I lost my taste for it. I had a fantastic filet mignon a couple of years ago, and I didn't like it.

People also often ask me whether this healthy lifestyle costs more than some may be able to afford. I have found, actually, that eating a healthy diet costs less than eating a poor diet. It costs a lot more to make yourself sick. People regularly tell me that they cut their food budgets in half by improving their diets. Organic fruits, vegetables, beans, grains and unprocessed oils may be more expensive than their nonorganic counterparts, but in the end a diet made up of healthful foods is cheaper. Consider what you pay for organic whole grains per pound versus what you pay for packaged breakfast cereal per pound, and you will realize quickly that unhealthful processed foods are much more expensive. Deadly, make-believe foods like ice cream, cola drinks and potato chips are expensive, provide little nutrition and damage your cells. Not purchasing them saves your money and your health. Even when a healthful choice does cost more, the purchase is well worth the investment because being sick is *very* expensive. The same holds true for supplements. The most expensive supplement of all is one that doesn't work, no matter how little you pay for it. High-quality supplements cost more, but they deliver the most nutrients to your cells. Most cheap vitamins do nothing, or almost nothing, and many contain toxins; many vitamin products cause both deficiency and toxicity.

Another important investment in health is to spend a little more on personal care and home-care products that do not harm your body. In making selections of toothpaste, shampoo, deodorants, skin creams and cosmetics, the most important criterion is that your body not be harmed. Selecting organic foods is not good enough; you must also select safe products. *If a product cannot be ingested without poisoning you, then it is not safe enough to put on your skin or your hair or your teeth.* Look at the swallowing warnings on a typical tube of toothpaste. (Consult appendix C for safe brands of toothpaste and other products.) The sad truth is that most personal-care products are toxic; those toxins bioaccumulate in your body and cause disease.

Look at Your Health in a New Way

The perspective we have to change is the way we look at and evaluate our own health. If you are going to solve your own health problems, you must first acknowledge they exist. We all grow up thinking that health is a given, until we "get sick." Rather than being static, however, health is a sliding scale, and our position and direction on that scale can change on a daily basis. This is why we need to learn how to evaluate our own health, in a meaningful and ongoing way, so as to avoid letting ourselves deteriorate to the point where we become sick.

As I was gradually losing my health, no one told me I was sick. In fact, I was told the opposite. At my periodic physical exams my physicians pronounced me in perfect health, even though I had required many fillings in my teeth and I suffered from a serious immune deficiency disease, namely from a seasonal allergy called "hay fever." Each year I suffered from one or more colds and every several years from a bout of flu. I was led to believe, however, that tooth decay, colds, flu and allergies are all normal and that I was healthy.

The fact is no one should have tooth decay, colds, flu, allergies or any other disease. If you do have any of these problems, you are experiencing substantial amounts of cellular malfunction and you are sick. Living with even that amount of cellular malfunction shortens your life and makes you susceptible to a host of other disease problems. Unless you do something different, your health will only get worse with time, not better. *Health cannot be improved by continuing to do the same things that made you sick.* Now is the time to make health your responsibility.

How to Read the Warning Signs

We all need to learn how to read the body's signals so that we can evaluate our own health and health decline. *Our body tells us when it is having trouble; our problem is that we don't listen.* Subtle signals are ignored until the problem becomes serious enough to demand attention.

How healthy are you? Often the warning signs are evident in your appearance; simply put, you don't look well. In addition, you should ask yourself whether you are experiencing

- Fatigue
- Aches and pains
- Skin problems
- Allergies
- Digestion troubles
- Sleep difficulties
- Susceptibility to infections
- Weight issues
- Mood, thought or behavior problems

These warning signs appear in ways that are usually easily recognized. Consider individually the signs listed.

Appearance

The body gives off visual signals, and we can learn to recognize them. I remember once seeing a friend and thinking, *He doesn't look well.* Not long thereafter, he was diagnosed with brain cancer. How many times have we looked at others and realized that they didn't look well? Before I took sick, my family thought I looked pale. Are you pale? Are there dark circles under your eyes? Are there wrinkles on your face? Is your hair graying? How well do you move? Are you well-coordinated? Are your eyes dull? Appearance matters, it is easy to check, and it should be checked on a regular basis.

Energy Level

Fatigue is probably the most common complaint made to doctors in our society because energy production at the cellular level is one of the first things affected as our cells malfunction and become diseased. If you do not have the energy you used to have, aging is not the problem. You are getting sicker.

Remember the boundless energy that healthy people like the Hunzas had? They performed physical feats such as traveling sixty miles in one day on foot, in mountainous terrain, and returning looking as though they had gone for a casual walk. Contrast this to the fatigue so many of us feel during the day, perhaps needing several cups of coffee just to keep going. Even many of our teenagers struggle with fatigue.

Skin Problems

Our skin is a barometer of overall health, but we are taught to think of a skin problem as just that, a skin problem. This is outmoded. Like any disease, skin problems are the result of systemic cellular malfunction. We may notice it in the skin, but the problem is likely affecting every cell in the body. The proper solution is not to use products like a cortisone ointment, but to restore the cells to good health. If your skin is dry, flaky, irritated, itchy, thin, has lost its elasticity, or if you develop skin lesions of any kind, you are not healthy.

Allergies

Allergies are not normal, and they do long-lasting damage to the body. Enhancing the health of your cells can eliminate allergies. Millions of Americans suffer from runny noses, sneezing, itching of the eyes, sinus problems, headaches, abdominal pain, diarrhea, skin rashes and numerous other problems as a result of allergies and sensitivities to foods, pollens, chemicals and other substances in our environment. We tend to look upon these reactions as "benign" inconveniences rather than the symptoms of a body out of balance. Allergies should be looked upon as a serious acquired immune dysfunction syndrome and treated by improving cellular health and strengthening the immune system.

Do you sneeze, develop a runny nose or have itchy eyes after eating a meal? Are your fingers sometimes swollen so that it is difficult to take off or put on a ring? Do you get loose stools after eating certain foods? All of these and more can be symptoms of allergic reactions. A body with allergies is not crying out for over-the-counter or prescription antihistamines, but for solving the problems of cellular malfunction. Like any other "disease," allergies can be both prevented and reversed by restoring normal function to the cells in your immune system. By working to minimize the deficiency and toxicity of my cells, I went from being allergic to virtually everything—called a "universal reactor"—to living a normal life.

Digestion Troubles

Do you have problems such as indigestion, inability to eat a wide variety of foods, intestinal cramps, abdominal bloating, excess gas, diarrhea, constipation, acid reflux, low energy, slow wound healing, or difficulty concentrating and thinking quickly and clearly? Good digestion is a foundation for achieving peak performance and optimal health. Yet digestive problems are epidemic in our society and they prevent millions of people from living the healthy, productive lives they would like. Most of our digestive problems are the direct result of poor diets, toxic exposure, lack of exercise, unresolved stress, and over-the-counter and prescription drugs. Digestive problems are more serious than people imagine, for *if you are not properly digesting your food and assimilating its nutrients, you will get sick, guaranteed.* Poor digestion is a perfect prescription for deficiency and toxicity, the two causes of disease.

Heartburn, bloating, gas and other digestive problems should not just be treated by antacids and other medications, and then forgotten. These problems are a wake-up call that one of our major body systems is not working right. A better solution is to chew your food well, do proper food combining, stay away from foods you are allergic to, take probiotics and digestive enzymes, and exercise regularly. Antibiotics may be the leading cause of digestive problems, and these dangerous drugs should be avoided for that reason alone.

Sleep Difficulties

Sleep is critical to health, but few of us sleep an adequate amount, and a growing number of people suffer from various sleep disorders, such as disturbed sleep patterns and insomnia. Much of the time sleep problems are symptoms that the hormones and chemicals the body uses to cope with stress are being depleted. The physical consequences of inadequate sleep have a negative effect on health and performance.

Healthy people like the Hunzas went to bed when it got dark and woke up with the sun. Try to go to bed at the same time every night and wake up at the same time every morning, even on weekends. Giving the body adequate and regular rest is important to maintaining good health.

Susceptibility to Infection

Colds and flu are not just inconveniences; they are alarm bells telling us that all is not well. While seen as a minor illness, each cold does permanent damage to the body, causing us to age prematurely. Yet millions of Americans suffer four to six colds per year, sometimes taking weeks to resolve. Healthy people do not get infections, and, if they do, they recover from them very quickly. You may recall that the healthy Hunzas never suffered from colds, and that the 133-year-old man in Vilcabamba had suffered only several colds in 133 years, not several in one year as many of us do. A cold or flu that lingers is further proof of widespread cellular malfunction. *If people around you are sick, worry about strengthening your own immunity, not about hiding from germs.* Building immunity is a long-term project; reacting in an emergency situation when you feel sickness coming on is something else. Here are ideas of how to accomplish both:

To prevent colds, take plenty of vitamin C (4,000 to 6,000 mg/day). If you are sick already, take vitamin C to bowel tolerance, which means taking it up to the point where you begin getting excessive gas or diarrhea and then backing off. Bowel tolerance will differ depending on who you are and what your state of health is. If I feel a cold coming on, I put 3,000 mg of vitamin C in a glass of water and drink it down every thirty to sixty minutes. In a matter of hours, the cold will be gone. B-vitamins are important, as are zinc and high-quality cod liver oil. Olive leaf extract can also be helpful; it is a powerful natural antibiotic. And, of course, avoid damaging your immunity with sugar, white flour, poor digestion, prescription drugs or anything that you are allergic to.

Weight Problems

Some people think being overweight is more of a fashion concern than a serious disease. Many people attribute weight problems to "genetics," saying that such problems run in their family. The truth is that being overweight is a sign that cells are malfunctioning. Often, an addiction to sugar is part of the problem, and this problem needs to be treated like any other addiction. Proper diet and lifestyle changes that improve cellular health are virtually guaranteed to solve weight problems. Overweight patients need to heal their cells, just like cancer patients and heart disease patients. Worse, weight problems are frequently the prelude to more serious chronic diseases.

Mood, Thought or Behavioral Problems

The ability to think quickly and clearly—to concentrate, learn and remember—are the benefits of healthy cells and a healthy body. A problem with any of these indicates deficiency and toxicity at the cellular level, usually the result of inappropriate diets, environmental toxins, lack of exercise and unresolved stress. Brain cells function normally when they have all the nutrition they need and do not have toxins that interfere with them.

The person who flies off the handle with little provocation is often seen as having a particular personality type. The same for those who have problems getting along with others or working out conflicts in a calm and rational manner. Most of the time, however, these problems point back to the same two causes of disease: deficiency and toxicity. We are currently experiencing an unprecedented epidemic of depression, learning disabilities, violent behavior and other types of mental disease. Many of these "mental" problems actually result from the fact that the function of our brains and nervous systems has never been more compromised. Worse, physicians usually try to "solve" these problems by giving those afflicted toxic, mind-altering chemicals.

Building a Better You

Now that you have a sense of your state of health and have perhaps identified some early warning signs of disease, start to build the foundation of a new lifestyle:

- Keep a food diary for a week, writing down everything you eat and drink. How much of your diet is eaten raw? Do you buy truly fresh, organic vegetables and fruits? Is the meat you eat treated with antibiotics and hormones? Do sugar, white flour, dairy products and processed oils bog down your diet? Do you combine the wrong foods together at a meal? Is the food you buy genetically modified?
- Keep track of the amount and kind of exercise, movement, or other physical stimulation (saunas, etc.) you participate in during the week.
- Consider the products you use on your body: Are the ingredients in your deodorant, toothpaste, shampoo, makeup and skin cream natural and nontoxic?
- Take a look at the products you use to clean your house. Consider, too, the furnishings, including your rugs. List the sources of emissions within your house, including your carpets, furnace, hot-water heater and stove.
- Consider the ways in which social connections, work and community involvement nurture you, or fail to do so.
- Take stock of the stress in your life.
- Think about the doctors you visit, the treatments or tests that you approve of, the medicines that you take. Are they doing you more harm than good? Are your doctors and your medical treatments addressing all your pathways to health, or is their focus narrow and incomplete?

- Do you take vitamins or other supplements consistently, and are they of high quality? Do they contain cheap, ineffective ingredients such as carbonates and oxides, or toxins such as artificial colors?

Each of these choices is part of an ongoing process of promoting—or antagonizing—your health. Keep track of all six pathways and do your best along each of them, all the time. Doing a great job for a week and then forgetting about it is pointless. Track the process—there is no endgame, no checkmate to seek—there is only process. *Either you are going about the process of getting well and staying well, or you are going about the process of getting sicker.* Keep trying new things until you discover what works for you.

After you have identified some of the problems in your lifestyle—ways in which your body is becoming deficient or ways in which toxins threaten you—begin today to make changes.

- Make sure at least some and preferably most of your diet is eaten raw. Buy at least some organic fresh fruits and vegetables, as well as organically produced meat. Cut down or eliminate the Big Four: sugar, white flour, dairy products and processed oils.
- Practice tips for proper food combining and effective food preparation methods to ensure you are getting the best nutrition from the food that you buy.
- Begin taking high-quality nutritional supplements.
- Make exercise and movement a part of every day.
- Nurture your social and family connections. Make a plan and then make a concerted effort to make it happen.
- Identify the drugs you take (medical or recreational), and begin to imagine how well you might function without them.

A Radical Shift in Perspective

As you consider your lifestyle and identify the areas that must change, take a close look at your overall perspective on health and disease. Health is something we all want, yet so few of us give it serious thought until we get sick. That approach does not work. The practical new system for choosing health presented in this book is different from typical approaches. This new way to "see" health and disease is so simple it empowers the individual to take charge. That empowerment can help to end our current epidemic of chronic and degenerative disease, dramatically improving the health of our people.

As I have told you, one of the first people whose perspective I helped change was my brother, diagnosed in 1991 with advanced prostate cancer. The specialist who made the diagnosis informed him that the tumor was so large and so widespread that surgery was not an option. My brother was told that there were no traditional medical treatment options available for his advanced stage of tumor. "Modern medicine" had nothing to offer, and my brother felt he was doomed. He eventually found a caring physician who was willing to operate, despite the poor odds. The surgery was a success, with limitations, as the surgeon was unable to remove all of the cancer, and biopsies indicated cancer had spread throughout my brother's body. His life expectancy was estimated between six months and three years, and no one in his condition had been known to live beyond five years.

As I am writing this chapter, eleven years have passed since my brother's surgery. He is living a high-quality life. How did he do it? First, he had to change his perspective. The existing belief system said he should have died a long time ago. Rather than accept his cancer as a death sentence, my brother took on the challenge of restoring normal function to his cells. The new understanding of one disease says disease has only two causes—deficiency and toxicity—and that addressing those causes along the six pathways can heal virtually all disease.

My brother's recovery came as the result of radical changes in diet and the addition of vitamin supplements, essential fatty acids and frozen shark cartilage—not chemotherapy and radiation. Conventional cancer treatments do nothing to reverse the underlying causes of cancer (abnormal cell chemistry), and they do devastating damage to the body.

The most important steps you can take to change your perspective about health, and thereby reduce morbidity and mortality, is to shift your view from one side of these equations to the other. That is, reconsider the differences between

- Disease care versus health care
- Diagnosing symptoms versus preventing disease
- Treating symptoms versus restoring health
- Relying on doctors versus relying on yourself
- Eating make-believe food versus eating real food
- Germs causing infection versus compromised immune systems
- Toxic versus nontoxic living
- An active life versus sedentary sickness

Let us take a closer look at each of these shifts in perspective.

Disease Care Versus Health Care

Existing medical practice is not about health care; it is about disease care. Modern medicine is based on the belief that you are healthy until you have a diagnosable disease, after which the task is to give the disease a name (diagnose) and then suppress (treat) its symptoms. This perspective waits for disease to happen; makes no attempt to measure health in its initial decline; ignores the effects of nutrition, toxins and behavior; and gives little or no recognition to the body's self-healing abilities. The patient is not empowered, and the personal and monetary costs are enormous. Modern medicine excels at treating emergencies and trauma, and in doing surgery, but does poorly at preventing or healing disease because it is almost totally unequipped to diagnose and treat the two causes.

The new perspective on health presented in this book is based not on waiting for disease to happen, but, rather, actively working to prevent disease. If disease does occur, then we must look for the true cause and restore health by addressing that root cause. This approach recognizes the body as self-regulating and self-healing, and seeks to optimize health by helping the body to function as it is designed to do. This approach incorporates all we have learned about the effects of nutrition, toxicity and behavior. The underlying inspiration is that health is a choice and that almost all disease is preventable.

Diagnosing Symptoms Versus Preventing Disease

The process of diagnosing a patient rests on waiting for illness to strike and then matching the symptoms to a so-called disease, thus giving that group of symptoms a category and a name. This activity can be very expensive and time consuming, and is often hazardous to the patient. Yet, what does it achieve? Does this tell us what caused the problem or how to fix it? Not very often. Because only one disease exists, spending a lot of time, money and resources to give a group of symptoms any one of thousands of meaningless names is not a productive activity.

Because of its focus on diagnosing and treating disease after it occurs, modern medicine has paralyzed itself, which is why it cannot reverse our epidemic of chronic disease. We cannot continue to perceive disease as something that strikes like a bolt of lightning; people in good health do not become ill. The only way to reduce disease is to promote health and thereby prevent disease in the first place.

Treating Symptoms Versus Restoring Health

The best way to deal with any problem—in business, personal lives, engineering, etc.—is to identify the cause, address the cause and solve the problem. Unfortunately, modern medicine does not focus on identifying the cause.

Traditional medicine suppresses symptoms, usually by poisoning patients with toxic drugs, removing essential body parts or exposing the patient to cancer-causing radiation—sometimes, all three tactics. Meanwhile, diseases remain chronic, and disease-care costs continue to escalate to unsustainable levels. *Diseases are healed with nutrients and the removal of toxins, not with drugs and surgical scalpels.*

Relying on Doctors Versus Relying on Yourself

Most people wait until they get sick, then go to a doctor and hope to get well. I did this when I was ill, only to discover that my physicians had no idea how to make me well. This practice negates our own responsibility for health. Do we really think we can eat an unhealthful diet and live an unhealthful lifestyle and that our doctor will make us well after we have worked so hard to make ourselves sick?

Health and disease are choices. We, as a society and as individuals, are the ones making those choices. Today, health is compromised at so many levels. If we want to improve our health, prevent or reverse disease, and extend life, we have to make special choices in order to compensate. We cannot rely on physicians to "fix" us after we have spent decades making ourselves sick—almost all physicians are stuck in the old disease-care paradigm and have no idea how to restore cells to health.

The responsibility for health is ours, and we must teach this to our children so they and their children can claim their birthright to lifelong good health. We must also ask our governments and society at large to make changes. Why do we allow soft drink and candy vending machines into our schools? Why is it that medical insurance covers failed traditional treatments but does not cover alternative treatments that are safer and more effective? Why do we allow our government to subsidize the dairy and sugar industries? Why do we allow genetically modified foods to be sold without labeling and without adequate testing for safety? Why do we continue to allow the use of fluoride in our drinking water? Why do we continue to allow dentists to put mercury in people's mouths? All of us need to address these questions and many others.

Eating Make-Believe Food Versus Eating Real Food

Until I educated myself, I used to think that what I purchased at the supermarket was real food. What a surprise to find little or no real food in a supermarket. Imagine the public outcry if someone had announced to us that they were going to drastically lower the nutritional content of our food. Yet, this is exactly what has happened. Where is the outcry? We are all eating nutritionally deprived, toxic, make-believe foods that have been proven incapable of supporting healthy life in either animals or humans.

Throughout this book we have looked at the history of the human diet and environment and how dramatically these have changed, especially in the last century. Our cells are designed with specific nutritional needs that are no longer satisfied by typical modern diets and lifestyles. To achieve optimal health, we must acquire daily all the nutrients for which we have genetic requirements. Scientist Linus Pauling, a Nobel laureate, wrote that modern diets are incapable of supplying optimal nutrient quantities, even if we make good food choices. According to eminent scientist Emanuel Cheraskin, M.D., D.M.D., up to 80 percent of the U.S. population suffers from malnutrition. Most of us now suffer from "affluent malnutrition," caused by an expensive diet rich in calories (from sugar and white flour) and poor in nutrients. Because the food supply is unhealthful, and has been for several generations, we are now seeing entire populations where no real perspective of "health" exists. Disease has become the norm, so we view ourselves as healthy.

Entire populations are now suffering from diseases that are unquestionably related to nutritional deficiency, yet we do not label them as such. This is because we seldom encounter obvious deficiency diseases such as scurvy, pellagra or beriberi, so malnutrition is not perceived as a major contributor to disease—but it is!

Deficiency in modern diets creates a host of problems including: diminished overall competence and resistance to infection, premature aging, colds and flu, acne, tooth decay, mental illness, heart disease, cancer, osteoporosis, kidney disease, lung disease, autoimmune disease, anemia, diabetes, allergies, birth defects, alcoholism, learning disabilities, violent behavior and more. Although these problems carry different disease labels, they are all the result of sick cells. Which body parts get sick does not matter, because the way to prevent disease or restore health is always the same. Give your cells what they need, protect them from what they don't need.

Nearly all supermarket fruits and vegetables have been grown in depleted soils and are deficient in nutrients and high in toxic contaminants. These substandard foods are often harvested before ripening so they can be shipped and stored without spoilage. Foods are often chemically enhanced to increase shelf life. A huge part of our diet has been processed and packaged, removing what little nutrition ever existed.

Does anyone really think that a donut made of white flour and sugar and soaked in rancid oils is real food? Real food is organic, fresh, raw, unprocessed and mainly plant-based. White flour, sugar, milk, ice cream and coffee are not real foods, nor are conventionally grown and prematurely harvested tomatoes, oranges and bananas, not to mention old, waxed apples and cucumbers. To prevent disease or to restore health, we must stop eating the make-believe and go back to what our healthy ancestors ate: real food.

Germs Versus the True Cause of Disease

The popular misconception is that microorganisms (germs) cause infections. But to be a true cause, the microorganisms would have to produce the same effect all the time, which is not the case. Not everyone who is exposed to a particular organism gets sick, and not everyone who gets sick does so to the same degree. In truth, whether or not someone develops an infection depends on the balance between several factors, namely the virulence of the organisms, the number of organisms and, most importantly, their state of immunity. We live in a sea of microorganisms, but they do not make us sick until we alter the natural balance between them and us. Our normal coexistence with germs rather than a germ-free environment ensures our health.

When we eat sugar and nutrient-deficient diets, expose ourselves to toxins, lose sleep, fail to exercise and fail to adapt to stress, our immunity becomes depressed and we open the door to infection. Then we blame the germ, when really we are to blame. Rather than being obsessed with germs and rushing for flu shots and antibacterial soaps, optimizing our immunity would be a far better approach. The perspective that germs cause disease is so ingrained in us, many have difficulty making the shift to the new way of thinking; but to avoid infection, we must do exactly that. People such as the Hunzas lived into their hundreds without ever having as much as a cold, not because they took flu shots but because they were healthy and their immune systems were strong. In truth, only sick people get sick. The problem is we spend decades making ourselves sick, all the while thinking we are healthy.

Toxic Versus Nontoxic Living

Imagine what would happen if someone announced that they were planning to poison our food, our homes, our workplaces or, for that matter, the entire planet? We would be outraged. Yet that has happened and few are outraged. We are constantly told that small amounts of toxins are safe. Yet chronic disease is rampant because these small amounts of toxins, when added together, are disabling our detoxification systems, exceeding our capacity to detoxify them, and bioaccumulating in our tissues to disease-causing levels.

Some toxins, such as estrogenic chemicals from pesticides, plastic bottles and canned foods, are not safe even in amounts so small they cannot be measured by the usual techniques. Every day we eat food, breathe air and use products containing these and other harmful toxins. Some exposure is virtually unavoidable, but most exposure is a choice. We have to start making different everyday choices about what we put on and in our bodies and what we expose ourselves to in the workplace. What we eat, wear and bring into our homes—and the personal care products that we use—are under our direct control. We need to change our perspective that small amounts of toxins are safe; we need to recognize that small amounts of toxins can build up in our bodies over time. Most Americans are now accumulating hundreds of man-made chemicals in their bodies, and yet we wonder why we get sick.

An Active Life Versus Sedentary Sickness

Human genes evolved at a time when a high level of physical activity was the norm. All through the course of evolution, man had to be physically active in order to survive. Our hunter-gatherer ancestors were nomadic peoples who were always on the move, always foraging for food or drink. Because of the way we evolved, the human body actually requires a high level of physical activity in order to function normally. Until fairly recently this activity requirement was met by leading a normal lifestyle and producing life's necessities. From prehistoric times up until the last century, people spent the vast majority of their physical energy—hard, daily labor—just trying to produce food, shelter and clothing. Today we are the most sedentary people in history. To achieve health, we must change our perspective that we can be both sedentary and healthy. Fortunately, for all you couch potatoes out there, a simple way is available to address this problem: rebounding. See appendix C for more information.

The Future Is Now

After bringing myself back from the brink of death and restoring my health, and after more than sixteen years of study and experimentation, I have concluded that the only way our society will stop its slide into declining health is to change our beliefs about health and disease. The next major advance in health care will be driven by those people who accept personal responsibility for their health, educate themselves and make choices that move their personal health equations away from disease and toward health.

When a large number of people look at something in the same way, we call that system of belief a paradigm. Paradigms become accepted wisdom, and we interpret our lives and make our decisions according to that conventional thinking. I ask you to reconsider accepted wisdom and conventional thinking about health, disease and medicine. Reconsider whether the beliefs that guide your life are effective in solving your problems. Reconsider whether the decisions you make about your health—from foods to drugs to doctors—bring you health and happiness. Reconsider whether you are missing out on tremendous opportunities to be well and to live a longer, more vigorous life than you ever imagined.

Today, most of us, and almost all of our physicians, are

living in a cave of confusion and misunderstanding. The medical establishment wins honors, praise and prizes for its descriptions of diseases and how to manage symptoms. Yet this health paradigm—this distorted way of viewing health—is not solving our problems.

If we are taught that thousands of diseases exist, then of course we must go to doctors for all our health problems; only the doctor has the education to deal with all the different diseases and their treatments. The new perspective I offer you is that there is only one disease; health is then easier to understand, and the power to get healthy and to stay healthy lies within yourself. Aside from medical emergencies, which are indeed matters for trained professionals, maintaining your health is a matter of preventing deficiency and toxicity and requires little or no outside assistance.

We like to think of ourselves as so technologically advanced, so smart, so sophisticated . . . able to invent computers, land on the moon and build space stations. Yet people we consider primitive lived much longer and healthier lives than we do. By optimizing their six pathways and minimizing the two causes of disease, these populations showed us that the potential for human health is extraordinary. These people did not suffer from the chronic and degenerative diseases that are the norm in our society; in fact they rarely, if ever, suffered from the common cold.

A massive misconception in America is that most of us are healthy. In reality, most of us are sick. You don't have to look sick to be sick. We are living proof that it is entirely possible to achieve normal growth rates and have a healthy appearance while being undernourished and in a state of compromised health. Our unprecedented epidemic of chronic and degenerative disease is clearly the result of eating a diet consisting of adulterated and devitalized foods; exposure to the lethal effects of polluted air, water and food; and exposure to man-made electromagnetic radiation. Yet, as a society, we have failed to come to grips with this reality, partially because we are still stuck in the obsolete medical paradigm of the "germs and genes theory" of disease, and partially because powerful economic incentives exist to maintain the status quo.

Do we think we can continue to eat nutritionally deficient diets, diets rich in make-believe foods made from sugar, white flour and processed oils, diets that will not even sustain healthy life in rats, and still be healthy? Can we continue to live sedentary lifestyles when we know that physical activity is absolutely essential to health? Can we continue to use products that poison us with toxins that bioaccumulate in our tissues and cause cellular malfunction? Can we support wellness without learning stress-management techniques? Can we continue to live and work in ways that deprive us of healthy, full-spectrum light and adequate sleep?

Chronic diseases such as cancer, heart disease, hypertension, diabetes, arthritis, asthma, allergies and osteoporosis are entirely preventable. By learning and universally applying the concepts of one disease, two causes and six pathways, our society could eliminate today's epidemic of chronic disease. We must teach everyone, including our schoolchildren, how to understand and take personal responsibility for the two causes of disease and how to form the positive habits that will result in lifelong good health. Health is a choice. Disease is the result of poor choices, and almost all diseases are preventable.

Throughout this book, you have learned the keys to a long and healthy life: perspective, power and perseverance. Understanding my theory of disease brings you a new perspective on health and modern medicine. Using that knowledge creates the power to choose your destiny. Persevere with the right choices along all six pathways toward health, and you will never be sick again!

REFERENCES

Appleton, Nancy. *Kick The Sugar Habit.* (Garden City Park, NY: Avery Publishing Group), 1996.

Balfour, E. *The Living Soil.* (New York: Universe Books), 1976.

Beasley, J. D., and Swift, J. J. *The Kellogg Report.* (Annandale-on-Hudson, NY: The Institute of Health Policy and Practice/Bard College Center), 1989.

Becker, R. O. *The Body Electric.* (New York: Quill/William Morrow), 1985.

Brekhman, I. I. and Nesterenko, I. F. *Brown Sugar and Health.* (New York: The Pergamon Press), 1983.

Casdorph, Richard and Walker, Morton. *Toxic Metal Syndrome.* (Garden City Park, NY: Avery Publishing Group), 1995.

Cheraskin, E., Ringsdorf, W. M., Jr., and Sisley, E. L. *The Vitamin C Connection.* (New York: Bantam Books), 1983.

Chopra, Deepak. *Ageless Body Timeless Mind.* (New York: Harmony Books), 1993.

Chopra, Deepak. *Creating Health.* (Boston, MA: Houghton Mifflin), 1987.

Chopra, Deepak. *Quantum Healing.* (New York: Bantam Books), 1989.

Cohen, A. M.; Bavly, S.; Poznanski, R. "Change of Diet of Yemenite Jews in Relation to Diabetes and Ischaemic Heart Disease." *The Lancet* (1961) 2:1399-1401.

Cohen, Robert. *Milk The Deadly Poison.* (Englewood Cliffs, NJ: Argus Publishing), 1997.

Coulter, Harris. *Vaccination, Social Violence and Criminality: The Medical Assault on the American Brain.* (Berkeley, CA: North Atlantic Books), 1990.

Cousins, Norman. *Anatomy of an Illness.* (New York: Bantam Books), 1979.

Crossing the Quality Chasm: A New Health System for the 21st Century. (Washington, D.C.: National Academy Press), 2001.

Cummins, Ronnie and Lilliston, Ben. *Genetically Engineered Food.* (New York: Marlowe & Company), 2000.

Dadd, Debra Lynn. *Nontoxic & Natural.* (Los Angeles, CA: Jeremy P. Tarcher, Inc.), 1984.

Diamond, Harvey. *Fit For Life: A New Beginning.* (New York: Kensington Books), 2000.

Ensminger, Aubrey, et al. *Food and Nutrition Enclycopedia.* (Clovis, CA: Pegus Press), 1983.

Erasmus, Udo. *Fats and Oils.* (Vancouver, Canada: Alive Books), 1986.

Erasmus, Udo. *Fats That Heal Fats That Kill.* (Burnaby, Canada: Alive Books), 1993.

Ershoff, B. H. "Synergistic Toxicity of Food Additives in Rats Fed a Diet Low in Fiber." *Journal of Food Science* (1976) 41:949-51.

Foster, Harold. "Lifestyle Changes and the Spontaneous Regression of Cancer: An Initial Computer Analysis." *International Journal of Biosocial Research,* vol. 10, no.1, p.17, (1988).

Goldberg, Burton et al. *Alternative Medicine: the Definitive Guide.* (Tiburon, CA: Future Medicine Publishing), 1993.

Gofman, John. *"Radiation from Medical Procedures in the Pathogenesis of Cancer and Ischemic Heart Disease: Dose Response Studies with Physicians Per 100,000 Population."* (San Francisco, CA: Committee for Nuclear Responsibility Books), 1999.

Gunderson, E. *"FDA Total Diet Study, April 1982–April 1986: Dietary Intakes of Pesticides, Selected Elements, and Other Chemicals."* (Arlington, VA: Association of Official Analytical Chemists), 1986.

Haley, Daniel. *Politics in Healing.* (Washington, D.C.: Potomac Valley Press), 2000.

Hoffman, Jay. *HUNZA: Secrets of the World's Healthiest and Oldest Living People.* (Clinton, NJ: New Win Publishing), 1997.

Internal Medicine News & Cardiology News, Consultatus Interruptus, December 1, 1993, page 9.

Jensen, Bernard. *Food for Healing Man.* (Escondito, CA: Bernard Jensen, Publisher), 1983.

Kaslow, A. L., and Miles, R. B. *Freedom from Chronic Disease.* (Los Angeles, CA: Tarcher), 1979.

Krohn, Jacueline and Francis Taylor. *Finding the Right Treatment.* (Point Roberts, WA: Hartley & Marks), 1999.

Lark, Susan, and Richards, James. *The Chemistry of Success.* (San Francisco, CA: Bay Books), 2000.

Lee, John R. *Optimal Health Guidelines.* (Sebastopol, CA: BLL Publishing), 1993.

Lee, John R. *Natural Progesterone.* (Sebastopol, CA: BLL Publishing), 1993.

Lewontin, Richard. *Human Diversity.* (New York: W. H. Freeman & Co.), 1982.

Lipski, Elizabeth. *Digestive Wellness.* (New Canaan, CT: Keats Publishing), 1996.

Lopez, D. A., M.D., Williams, R. M., M.D., and Miehlke, K., M.D. *Enzymes The Fountain of Life.* (Charleston, SC: The Neville Press), 1994.

McGee, C. T. *How to Survive Modern Technology.* (New Canaan, CT: Keats Publishers), 1979.

McTaggert, Lynne. *What Doctor's Don't Tell You.* (San Francisco, CA: Thorsons/Harper Collins), 1996.

Mead, Nathaniel. "Don't Drink Your Milk," Natural Health, July/August, 1994, 70.

Mendelsohn, R. S. *Confessions of a Medical Heretic.* (Chicago, IL: Contempoary Books), 1979.

Murphy, Suzanne et al. "Demographic and economic factors associated with dietary quality for adults in the 1987–88 Nationwide Food Consumption Survey." *Journal of the American Dietetic Association,* Vol. 92, No. 11, November 1992.

New England Journal of Medicine, "Iatrogenic Illness on a General Medical Service at a University Hospital" (304–11) Mar. 12, 1981: 638-642.

Null, Gary. *Get Healthy Now.* (New York: Seven Stories Press), 1999.

Ornstein, Robert and Sobel, David. *The Healing Brain.* (New York: Simon & Schuster), 1987.

Oski, Frank. *Don't Drink Your Milk.* (Brushton, NY: TEACH Services), 1983.

Ott, John. *Health and Light.* (Columbus, OH: Ariel Press), 1976.

Pauling, Linus. *How to Live Longer and Feel Better.* (New York: Avon Books), 1986.

Pearce, Joseph. "Nutrition Beliefs: More Fashion Than Fact." *FDA Consumer,* June 1976: 25-27.

Pfeiffer, Carl C. *Mental and Elemental Nutrients.* (New Canaan, CT: Keats Publishers), 1975.

Pottenger, F. M., Jr. *Pottenger's Cats.* (La Mesa, CA: Price-Pottenger Nutrition Foundation), 1983.

Quillin, Patrick. *Beating Cancer with Nutrition.* (Tulsa, OK: Nutrition Times Press), 1994.

Randolph, Theron and Moss, Ralph. *An Alternative Approach to Allergies.* (New York: Harper and Row), 1980.

Robbins, John. *Diet for a New America.* (Walpole, NH: Stillpoint Publishing), 1987.

Robinson, M. H. "On sugar and white flour . . . the dangerous twins!" in *A Physician's Handbook on Orthomolecular Medicine.* (Tarrytown, NY: Pergamon Press), 1977.

Rodale, J. I. *The Healthy Hunzas.* (Emmaus, PA: Rodale Press), 1949.

Rose, Steven. *Lifelines: Biology Beyond Determinism.* (New York: Oxford University Press), 1997.

Schneider, Meir et al. *The Handbook of Self-Healing.* (New York: Penguin Arkana), 1994.

Scheibner, Viera. *Vaccination.* (Blackheath, NSW: Australian Print Group), 1993.

Schoenthaler, Stephen, et al, "The Impact of a Low Food Additive and Sucrose Diet on Academic Performance in 803 New York City Schools," *International Journal of Biosocial Research,* 8(2), 1986, pg 185-195.

Schreiber, S. L. "Using the Principles of Organic Chemistry to Explore Cell Biology." *Chemical and Engineering News.* 22–32, October 26, 1992.

Schroeder, Henry. *The Poisons Around Us.* (New Canaan, CT: Keats Publishing), 1978.

Schwartz, Jack. *It's Not What You Eat But What Eats You.* (Berkeley, CA: Celestial Arts), 1988.

Simonton, O. C., Matthews-Simonton, S. and Creighton, J. L. *Getting Well Again.* (New York: Bantam Books), 1978.

Smith, Lendon. *Feed Yourself Right.* (New York: Dell Publishing), 1983.

Steinman, David. *Diet for a Poisoned Planet,* (New York: Random House, Inc.), 1990.

Steinman, D. and Epstein, S. S. *The Safe Shoppers Bible,* (New York: Macmillan), 1995.

Stitt, P. A. *Fighting the Food Giants.* 2nd Ed. (Manitowoc, WI: Natural Press), 1981.

Tesler, Eugene. "Nutrition and Eating: Do Americans Practice What They Preach?" *Food Product Development* June 1978: 82-86.

U.S. Office of Technology Assessment *Assessing the Efficacy and Safety of Medical Technologies,* Congress of the United States, 1978.

Vander, Arthur. *Nutrition, Stress, & Toxic Chemicals: An Approach to Environmental Health Controversies,* (Ann Arbor, MI: University of Michigan Press), 1981.

Walker, Morton *Secrets of Long Life.* (Old Greenwich, CT: Devin-Adair), 1983.

Williams, Roger J. *Nutrition Against Disease.* (New York: Bantam Books), 1971.

Williams, Roger J. *The Wonderful World Within You.* (Wichita, Kansas: Bio-Communications Press), 1977.

Yudkin, J. *Pure, White and Deadly. The Problem of Sugar.* Davis-Poynter, 1974.

AUTHOR'S NOTE: GOING BEYOND HEALTH

After deciding, in 1991, to devote the remainder of my life to helping others achieve health, I knew I needed to develop an approach that would eliminate all the confusion and misinformation. I needed to simplify health and disease. Next, I needed a model easily understood and applied by adults and children alike. My new theory of health and disease was born—One Disease, Two Causes and Six Pathways. The next need was to identify safe and effective products of all kinds, which would support health as indicated by the model.

In order for my work to benefit the public, I needed effective methods of presenting both my health model and my research. I needed people to understand the ineffectiveness of our society's current health model (medical suppression of disease symptoms). I also needed to demonstrate the significance of the damage we commonly suffer from seemingly benign sources (small amounts of toxins capable of bioaccumulating to dangerous levels in our bodies). Perhaps most important, I wanted to share what I had learned about the benefits of good nutrition and a healthful lifestyle.

My answer to these needs was to create a new entity called Beyond Health. My goal in creating Beyond Health was to help people achieve a level of vitality and performance surpassing anything they had experienced before—to help them go "beyond health." Today, Beyond Health is a unique resource for people who care about their health, providing two major services to the public: It supplies accurate, cutting-edge health information and makes available the world's best health-supporting products.

Unfortunately, there is a great deal of conflicting information, particularly with vitamin supplements and personal care products, and consumers remain confused about how to make the best choices. It is very difficult to know, merely by reading the label, if products are healthful and/or toxic. In my own recovery process, I had to be extremely careful about the products I selected. Even small amounts of impurities and toxins were enough to make me ill. I ended up with a refrigerator full of vitamin supplements that I could not take because of toxic contamination. I later realized that even healthy people were being injured by these same impurities and toxins, even though it may not be obvious to them. Beyond Health researches and approves only the safest and most effective choices in supplements, foods and personal products— discerning between those that claim to be the best and those for which there is credible evidence that they really are the best. This is a difficult, time-consuming and unique service.

Cutting through the contradictions and confusion, Beyond Health translates a chaotic mountain of medical and scientific data into the critical knowledge that people must have in order to maintain healthy bodies. This information is made available in several different ways, including public appearances at health conferences around the world, through my newsletter, *Beyond Health News,* and through my radio talk show, *An Ounce of Prevention.*

My latest venture is a nonprofit foundation, Health-e-America

Foundation (HeAF). HeAF's purpose is to end the epidemic of chronic disease in America by educating our schoolchildren about the basics of good health using the One Disease, Two Causes, Six Pathways model. For more information on Health-e-America Foundation see appendix F. For more information on the radio show and newsletter, see appendix A.

Finding the Needle in a Haystack

Perhaps a few examples will best illustrate the difficulty in discerning among the most healthful products and information. It took eighteen months of study and analysis to find a single brand of toothpaste that did not contain toxic ingredients (colors, flavors, fluoride or toxic foaming agents) but still cleaned teeth well. It took two years to find a safe and effective deodorant. It took eight months to find a pure and healthful brand of olive oil that contained only fresh, high-quality olives and was extracted in a manner that would neither damage the nutrients in nor create toxins in the oil. Recommendations for toothpaste, deodorant, olive oil, and other products can be found in appendix C.

Vitamin supplements were the biggest challenge. Almost half of all vitamin brands do not dissolve quickly enough to be of any use to the human body, and many do not contain all the nutrients listed on the label. Most brands contain cheap ingredients that have only marginal biological activity. *In fact, the vast majority of vitamin brands on the market are not worth what you pay for them—they are only marginally useful, and many contain toxins such as solvent residues and artificial colors.* It took me over a year of research to find a superior multivitamin brand and several additional years to find a superior brand of vitamin E (see appendix B for what I use and recommend in vitamin supplements).

It is amazing how many difficulties the average person faces in trying to make healthful choices. I find it a full-time job to keep up, but it is a job worth doing. I learned the hard way how suffering can come when health is failing; the challenge and success of recovering from a terminal illness has given me an opportunity to arrive at unique insights that I am now sharing with you.

Perhaps the most profound conclusions I reached in my study of health are that *health is a choice* and that *virtually no one ever has to be sick.* But first, we must educate ourselves; we must know not only what to look for, but how to look. To choose health, we must learn how to make better choices in the foods we eat, the supplements we take and the products we use.

While most of the products I selected for my own use are available in health food stores, some are not in every store or every state. To make life easy for those who care about their health, Beyond Health makes most of the products I use and recommend available to the public.

Beyond Health can be reached by calling 800-250-3063 or by accessing *www.beyondhealth.com.*

APPENDIX A
HEALTH INFORMATION

An Ounce of Prevention

A*n Ounce of Prevention* has been called the best health show in America. On the frontier of health information, this radio talk show will give you a regular supply of critical health knowledge. For information on how to access the *Ounce of Prevention* show on the air or the Internet, go to *www.beyondhealth.com.*

Beyond Health News

This bi-monthly, cutting-edge newsletter features the latest scientific breakthroughs and critical information essential to your health. We often bring you information that is years, sometimes decades, ahead of mainstream media and other health newsletters:

- The first in the world to warn the public of the cancer-causing danger of local anesthetics.
- The first, outside of Italy and Switzerland, to expose the scandal in the olive oil industry, and its negative health effects.

- Medical doctors supply reprints of our osteoporosis article to their patients.
- Groundbreaking articles on the health hazards of vaccinations, hormone replacement therapy, X rays, microwaved foods, and milk.

Tape Album

Never Be Sick Again—a double cassette album for those who want the principles of *Never Be Sick Again* the book on tape.

For more information go to *www.beyondhealth.com* or call 800-250-3063.

APPENDIX B
VITAMIN SUPPLEMENTS

Millions of Americans take vitamin supplements on a daily basis. Does it improve their health? For the most part, no. Large-scale epidemiological studies have been unable to find health benefits in those who take vitamins. Confused? There is a simple explanation. Most vitamin products are ineffective and even the best-selling brands contain toxins. Indeed, taking supplements will benefit your health, but only if you take the correct supplements.

After years of research and testing vitamin products, I selected the Perque brand for my own use. During my recovery from terminal illness, I knew I needed a nutritional supplement supply of the highest quality. Even small amounts of impurities and toxins were sufficient to make me very sick, thus *purity* was one of my most important criteria in choosing vitamins. As it turns out, fillers and/or chemical additives constitute about half of most vitamin brands. These fillers can introduce toxins and allergens, interfere with solubility and/or absorption and ultimately reduce the biological activity at the cellular level. Why bother to take a supplement if it's going to

contribute to your toxic load, or if the impurities will prevent
the nutrients from reaching and being metabolized inside the
cells?

Almost half of all vitamin brands do not dissolve soon
enough to be assimilated by the body. Even among brands that
dissolve soon enough, most of them provide only the RDA of
the nutrients they contain, yet it takes much more than the
RDA to be biologically significant in preventing or reversing
disease. Furthermore, just because a vitamin pill contains a
nutrient does not mean that the nutrient will be useful to your
body. Cheap and inappropriate raw materials (with low biological activity) are used most often in the major vitamin
brands. Some manufacturers even make a habit of purchasing
—at tremendous discounts—outdated raw materials that have
lost their potency. *The most expensive vitamin pill in the world
is one that doesn't work.*

It is neither easy nor cheap to make a quality vitamin product. Consider the question of synthetic versus naturally
derived vitamins. Natural ingredients tend to be more biologically available and more expensive, which is why most vitamin brands use synthetics. The molecules of these synthetics
often differ in shape from the natural molecules, which is
important in how they react, and thus how the body uses them.
For example, synthetic vitamin E and beta-carotene are well
known to be less biologically active than their natural forms.
Taking synthetic beta-carotene can even cause a deficiency of
other carotenes. In addition to the problems posed by synthetics, other considerations include the age and purity of the raw
materials and how they are shipped, stored, handled, compounded and packaged. All these can have a big effect on the
quality of the finished product.

Based on the criteria I set for safety, quality and effective-
ness, the one brand that stood out from the crowd was Perque.
In my weakened and chemically hypersensitive condition,
Perque was the first brand of supplement my body was able to

tolerate, especially at therapeutic doses. Only after taking Perque did my health begin to improve. These supplements are extraordinarily pure and have exceptionally high biological activity. The vitamin E brand I selected for my own use is called Unique E.

Unfortunately, because of the many subtleties and complexities, it is almost impossible for the consumer to make an informed judgment about the quality of a vitamin supplement. There is a great deal of information you need to know that simply cannot be found on the label. There are, however, some clues anyone can look for such as the chemistry of the minerals. If you find carbonates, oxides, sulfates, phosphates and chelates, you are most likely looking at an inferior formula. Save your money, because your cells will see little, if any, benefit. Also, a multivitamin containing iron, iodine or copper is not well designed because these can cause loss of antioxidant nutrients in the formula. A formula that lists beta-carotene without listing the source is most likely the inferior synthetic variety. Vitamin E with a "dl" in front of it is the less desirable synthetic version. The best solution is to research and understand the chemistry of the supplements thoroughly or else purchase from a trusted source.

Based on what your body actually gets for what you pay, Perque is the least expensive brand and the best value on the market, which is why I recommend it and use it myself. For more information about Perque and Unique E go to *www.beyondhealth.com* or call 800-250-3063.

APPENDIX C
FOODS AND PERSONAL
PRODUCTS

Most of the countless thousands of products on the market today do not meet my criteria for both safety and effectiveness. Many are effective, but fail on the safety issue. A few brands are in the acceptable category for use by most people. However, especially for those who have health problems and are struggling to get well, I recommend only those products that have met my standards for both effectiveness and safety. Following is a list of products I have chosen for my own use. Most of these are available at *www.beyondhealth.com* or by calling 800-250-3063.

Cleaning Cloth

Most household glass, bathroom, and kitchen cleansers contain toxic chemicals that are damaging to cells. The nontoxic answer is One Cloth. One Cloth cleans almost anything with just water, even greasy stoves and car windshields. Use a spray bottle with water instead of toxic chemicals. When a One Cloth gets dirty, just throw it in the regular wash (do not use chlorine bleach and they will last through hundreds of washings).

Deodorant

Most people use deodorants daily and are unaware that they are placing toxic chemicals on a sensitive skin area where they can be absorbed into the body. Almost all deodorants contain toxic chemicals such as aluminum compounds, triclosan, and artificial fragrances, colors and preservatives. Even the "rock" deodorants are made of aluminum salts. After two years of research, my choice is IndiuMagic. IndiuMagic is a colorless, odorless liquid spray that is non-staining, non-allergenic, safe, inexpensive and effective.

Fats and Oils

Certain fats and oils are essential nutrients. The body requires them every day for good health. The problem is that most of the good fats and oils have been removed from our modern diets and unhealthful fats and oils have replaced them. The fats and oils I choose to use follow.

Bariani Olive Oil

Most commercial olive oil is processed in a manner that damages its nutritional content. Most of the time people are *not* getting what they *think* they are buying when they purchase a bottle of olive oil (hence the scandal in the olive oil industry which was first introduced to the public by my newsletter, *Beyond Health News,* and was ultimately included in a worldwide broadcast by the BBC and by ABC news). Almost all olive oil is processed and diluted in ways that result in the loss of vitamins, essential fatty acids, antioxidants, and other nutrients, not to mention the addition/creation of toxins. In my search for a healthful olive oil, I found only one U.S. producer that's doing everything right. Not surprisingly, this oil also has the best flavor; the brand is Bariani.

Barleans Flaxseed Oil

Everybody needs essential fats. Flaxseed oil contains essential omega-3 and -6 fatty acids that are required for good health. In choosing an oil, look for one that is as fresh as possible and unfiltered, so as to retain all its precious nutrients and goodness. Barleans is my choice. It is a high-quality oil that is pressed daily, given a four-month shelf life date stamp and expressed directly to your local health food store.

Carlson Cod Liver Oil

Carlson Cod Liver Oil comes from the livers of fresh cod fish found in the pure North Atlantic waters near Norway. It is a rich source of vitamins A and D along with DHA and EPA (fish oils beneficial to human health).

Organic Ghee or Butter

Organic butter is acceptable when a fat is required, such as for frying. Do not allow the butter to smoke, as it becomes toxic. Organic ghee (clarified butter) may be a better choice since it lacks the milk proteins and is less allergenic than butter. Ghee is made by removing all the milk solids and water from butter, leaving only the fat. Ghee withstands higher temperatures well, making it ideal for cooking. My choice is Purity Farms Organic Ghee.

Udo's Choice Perfected Oil Blend

Udo's Choice is a blend of organic, unrefined oils and nutritional co-factors that balances the omega-3 and omega-6 fatty acids to coincide with those obtained from traditional diets.

Pesticides

Pesticides are among the most dangerous of all man-made chemicals. When we are exposed to pesticides, not only do they harm us and our children; they harm all life on the planet. Yet, there are times when it sure would be nice to have something that effectively kills and repels bugs without doing harm to you, your children, your pets, or the environment. I found such a product; it is called Orange Guard.

pH paper

pH balance is a critical part of cellular health. For monitoring the pH of urine and saliva, pH paper in the range of 5.5 to 8.0 is ideal. pH paper in this range is available at Beyond Health, along with guidelines on how to measure and control your pH.

Rebounding

Health is determined by many factors, including diet, toxins, genes, stress, thoughts and emotions and *the amount of physical activity we get*. Research has proven that the benefits of exercise are cumulative and that physical activity is essential for health. Rebounding is a simple, easy, and inexpensive way to address this problem without leaving your home.

If you consider buying a rebounder, do not purchase a cheap $50 mini-trampoline at your local sporting goods store. This type of rebounder actually can do more harm than good. Inexpensive rebounders tend to have bad springs; these cheap tube springs do not absorb and cushion your weight properly, causing a bounce that is abrupt and jarring. People have suffered permanent nerve damage from using such units. Select a rebounder with fat, barrel spring that allows for smooth deceleration, bringing you to a gentle stop. Another problem with cheap rebounders is poor-quality matting material. Cheap mats stretch too much, do not support your feet properly and thus place undue stress on your ankles, knees and back. By contrast, good rebounders have high-quality mats that hold their shape and do not overstretch. Other considerations for a rebounder include the strength of the frame, the height and number of legs, the quality of the sewing that attaches the webbing to the mat and the ease with which the unit can be folded, stored out of the way or made portable. The rebounder I selected for my personal use is available through Beyond Health.

Shampoo

All shampoos will remove oil and dirt from your hair, but the challenge is finding one without toxins. Common toxins include sodium lauryl sulfate and artificial colors, fragrances and preservatives. Depending on the formula, other ingredients in shampoo are capable of reacting with sodium lauryl sulfate to form nitrosamines, which are powerful carcinogens. The brand I chose for my personal use is Aubrey Organics. Aubrey makes a variety of shampoo products, so there is bound to be one that is just right for you.

Skin Cream

Like shampoos, most skin creams contain a long list of highly toxic chemicals including artificial colors, fragrances, and preservatives such as parabens (capable of damaging sublayers of skin even more severely than a bad sunburn—damage that goes essentially unnoticed—until a cancer diagnosis). My search for a skin cream that contained no toxins and only high-quality natural ingredients led me again to Aubrey Organics, which makes a variety of safe and effective skin creams. My favorite is their Green Tea & Ginkgo

Moisturizer, which is available at quality health and specialty stores or at Beyond Health.

Soap

Soaps generally come in either bar or liquid form and are made from either vegetable or animal fats or synthetic detergents. There are enormous differences in the amount of skin irritation caused by different brands of soap. Generally, soaps made from glycerin are among the mildest. Soaps can also contain a variety of toxins including artificial colors and fragrances as well as antibacterial chemicals. I look for soaps that minimize both skin irritation and toxicity while still doing the job. My favorites are soaps made by Weleda and Aubrey Organics. I also like Kirk's Castile bar soap and Dr. Bronner's liquid soaps; both are effective, safe and relatively inexpensive.

Sunscreen

This is a perspective issue more than a recommendation. Sunlight is a health promoting, required nutrient. Sunburn, however, damages health. The answer is to get sun in frequent moderate doses and build a tan. Unless you do something foolish, the sun will not cause disease in healthy people who have adequate amounts of nutrients like carotenes, lycopene, essential fatty acids, and vitamins A, C, E, and zinc and selenium. Our need for the sun is exemplified by the fact that nature intended us to get most of our vitamin D from the sun. Vitamin D is almost totally absent in vegetable foods. If you must have a sunscreen skin product, I recommend looking for those that do not contain any toxic, synthetic chemicals. My personal choices are any of the several sunscreen products by Aubrey Organics, or merely sticking to the ancient Mediterranean custom of rubbing high quality olive oil (such as Bariani) on the skin.

Synthetic chemical sunscreens may indeed help prevent a sunburn, but they do not prevent skin cancer—in fact, they may even promote it. Researchers at the M.D. Anderson Cancer Center in Houston cite: "There is no substantial evidence that sunscreen protects against any of the three forms of skin cancer." Robin Marks, M.B., M.P.H., a dermatologist and a professor at the University of Melbourne said: "Relying on synthetic chemicals to prevent cancer is laughable." Arthur Rhodes, a University of Pittsburgh dermatologist, told a 1994 meeting of the American Cancer Society that sunscreens "appear weakly effective or ineffective."

Toothpaste

Because almost all toothpaste is toxic, I looked for a toothpaste that would clean teeth without adding to toxic overload. The mucus membranes in the mouth are highly permeable and chemicals in toothpaste pass right through the membranes into the blood stream where they can bioaccumulate in the body to toxic levels. Toxins such as sodium lauryl sulfate, fluoride, artificial sweeteners, artificial colors, and artificial flavors are common contaminants in toothpaste. The brand I selected after eighteen months of research is Weleda. While there may be other acceptable brands, I did not find any in my search that were superior to Weleda. If you decide to look for one on your own, the objective is to find a brand that is made from only natural and exceptionally pure raw materials.

For additional information about these products, go to *www.beyondhealth.com* or call 800-250-3063.

APPENDIX D
ALTERNATIVE CANCER TREATMENTS

ancer may be the most feared of all diseases, but like all so-called diseases, it is nothing more than malfunctioning cells. Restore those cells to normal function and the cancer will disappear. Modern medicine's dangerous treatments have failed to put a dent in our cancer epidemic. Meanwhile, alternative methods have been clinically proven to reverse cancer.

Good resources include the *Definitive Guide to Cancer* by Diamond, Cowden, and Goldberg, published by Future Medicine Publishing. Another resource is *Beating Cancer with Nutrition* by Patrick Quillin. For specific suggestions regarding alternative treatment options, consult with People Against Cancer. By becoming a paid member, they will provide information about treatment options through an International Physicians Network that reviews your medical records and provides specific recommendations. In addition, People Against Cancer provides a wide range of educational materials of interest to people with cancer.

For more information go to *www.beyondhealth.com* and click on the links page or call 800-250-3063.

APPENDIX E
IMPROVING VISION

Eyesight can be improved using natural vision improvement exercises. By regularly performing a series of simple exercises, most people can throw their eyeglasses away. Meir Schneider's *Yoga for Your Eyes* offers a complete program including a 62-page booklet, eye exercise chart, and an 82-minute videotape teaching you how to improve your vision naturally. Meir Schneider was born without sight. He developed his own total approach to self-healing and used it to reverse his own blindness. *Yoga for Your Eyes* is available through Beyond Health at *www.beyond-health.com* or 800-250-3063.

APPENDIX F
HEALTH-E-AMERICA
FOUNDATION

D*ramatic increases in disease-care costs and rates of disease are threatening to overwhelm the economic and social structures of the United States.* An aging population and an unprecedented epidemic of chronic and degenerative disease are making costs spin out of control. With the percentage of young taxpayers shrinking, providing health benefits to the elderly will overwhelm the national budget within thirty years. The United States spends more on health care than any other nation. Yet the incidence of almost every chronic disease continues to increase, the health of our people continues to deteriorate, and costs are soaring to unsustainable levels. According to the Medicare Board of Trustees, Medicare spending will double over the next ten years. Medicare costs will exceed those of Social Security, and by 2030, 75 percent of the federal budget will be allocated to Medicare, Medicaid, and social security. The promised benefits under Medicare and social security are projected to exceed scheduled income by $465 trillion over the next 75 years.

The combined economic and social disruption from

supporting such a large, diseased population could be catastrophic. *A program to prevent this crisis must become a
national priority.*

The solution to this crisis is to arrest and reverse the epidemic, thereby lowering health costs to a fraction of today's
expenditures. Aging is inevitable, but health is a choice. The
variable over which we have control is whether people remain
healthy as they age. We must teach them how to do this. Since
this epidemic is man-made, we can choose to unmake it
through a dramatical and new scientifically based education
model.

The mission of Health-e-America Foundation (HeAF) is
to arrest and reverse our chronic-disease epidemic through
education—by teaching schoolchildren and their families the
basics of good health and empowering them to achieve it.
With childhood disease rates increasing, teaching children
how to improve health and avoid disease will produce an
almost immediate reduction in costs, with the savings compounded each year.

Health-e-America Foundation will provide health education
using a new model of health and disease based on the revolutionary concept of maintaining and improving cellular health.
In essence, there is only one disease—malfunctioning cells. It
is malfunctioning cells that become susceptible to infection
and which manifest as cancer or other so-called diseases.
Teaching children how to prevent and repair cellular malfunction will begin to immediately arrest and reverse America's
chronic disease epidemic. This epidemic took generations to
create, but we must reverse it much faster. This can only be
accomplished by teaching an entire generation of children.

Existing health education is disjointed and incomplete. It
has not been effective in curtailing this epidemic because it
fails to provide a coherent understanding of health. Worse,
most of the existing educational materials have been supplied
by industries promoting unhealthful or outmoded solutions.

The *one-disease concept* is a vastly more effective way to teach health. This concept is easy to understand and it is a comprehensive system incorporating all aspects of health. Using advanced E-learning technology, HeAF will provide, *free of charge* and in CD ROM format or online, educational materials that are stimulating to students and available to teachers in grades kindergarten through high school. HeAF will produce these unique educational materials as well as launch a national educational campaign for parents, teachers, and school administrators to facilitate the introduction and use of these materials in the schools. This program will benefit the existing generation, but most important, it will improve the health of each succeeding generation, which we all have a responsibility to ensure—to ensure the future of America.

For more information on HeAF go to *www.healtheamerica.org*. To support this important work, tax-deductible donations can be sent to:

Health-e-America Foundation
P.O. Box 150578
San Rafael, CA 94915

"Never doubt the power of small groups to change the world; indeed, it is the only thing that ever has."

Margaret Mead,
Anthropologist 1901–1978

INDEX

detoxification, 59, 147, 191–93
DHA (docosahexanoic acid),
104–5
DHEA, 304
diabetes, 18, 19, 21–22, 91, 92,
100, 102, 159
diagnosis, dying from, 207
diagnostic tests, 293
Diamond, Harvey, 90
dieldrin, 148–49
Diet for a New America
(Robbins), 105–6, 148
Diet for a Poisoned Planet
(Steinman), 106–7
diet
avoiding toxins in, 154
cause of declining health,
30–31
nutritionally deficient, 23
optimal, 28–29
dietary supplements, need for,
131–36
diets, 226
digestion, steps for, 123
digestion troubles, 327–28
digestive damage, 298–99
digestive destruction, 306–7
digestive enzyme supplements,
129
digestive toxins, 185–86
disease
causes of, xiv, 40, 44–46, 62,
339
chronic among U.S.
population, 20
defining, 43–44
diagnosable, 54

elimination of, 63
expectation of, 22
healing, 336
localized approach to,
281–82
one, xiv, 40, 43–44
preventable, 19, 335
problems not solved by
surgery, 294
reasons for, 19
rethinking, 341–43
as set of symptoms, 46–49,
279
simplifying, 42–50
susceptibility to, 50–56
disease care, vs. health care,
334–41
"diseases of aging," 18, 146
diseases of civilization, 146
diuretics, 278, 297
doctor strikes, death rates
declining during, 289
Don't Drink Your Milk, 100
Dossey, Larry, 215–16
Down's syndrome, 291
drug industry, 287–88
drugs, 81, 279
adverse reactions to, 296–97
cause of disease, 295–96
morbidity and mortality
costs related to, 297
over-the-counter, 20,
183–84, 280. *See also*
nonsteroidal anti-
inflammatory drugs